EPILEPSY
AND PREGNANCY

EPILEPSY AND PREGNANCY

What Every Woman with Epilepsy Should Know

Stacey Chillemi

and

Blanca Vazquez, M.D.

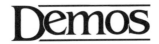

Demos Medical Publishing, LLC, 386 Park Avenue South, New York, New York 10016

Visit our website at www.demosmedpub.com

The purpose of this book is to provide information to readers so that they can make more informed decisions about their own health care. It should not be construed as medical advice and readers should always consult with their doctors.

Library of Congress Cataloging-in-Publication Data

Chillemi, Stacey. Epilepsy and pregnancy : what every woman with epilepsy should know / Stacey Chillemi and Blanca Vazquez.
    p. cm.
  Includes bibliographical references and index.
  ISBN 1-932603-15-8 (alk. paper)
  1. Epilepsy in pregnancy. I. Vazquez, Blanca. II. Title.
RG580.E64E63 2006
618.3'68—dc22

2005028356

Printed in Canada

I dedicate this book to my wonderful family: to my husband, Michael, who has *always* accepted me for who I am and supported me through my highs and lows, and to my children, Mikey, Alexis, and Anthony, whom I love with all my heart and soul. I am blessed to share my life with you. Thank you for being who you are, and for being by my side when I needed your love and support. Thank you for opening my eyes so that I might see the beauty of life in a whole different light.

Contents

Acknowledgments

I would like to convey a special thank-you to my parents for loving me unconditionally, for encouraging me to become a mother, and for giving me the love and support I needed before, during, and after my pregnancies.

I am also extremely grateful to Marie, my best friend, who has been there for me since we were kids. I would also like to convey my love and appreciation to my extended family and friends, who stood by me and supported me throughout the challenges of epilepsy.

Preface

I hope this book will help women with epilepsy who want to have children but are afraid to because of their disorder. Myths about epilepsy are still present in our society, and they generate unnecessary fear, preventing women with epilepsy from having children. There are many things any woman needs to consider when she wants to become pregnant, and this is especially true if you have epilepsy. This book will give women with epilepsy a better understanding of what to expect when they become pregnant, so that they can decide if motherhood is meant for them.

I also hope this book will help women with epilepsy who are currently pregnant and have questions that need to be answered. I had many fears and worries during my pregnancies, and I wanted to speak with someone who had gone through what I was going through, someone who could relate to me and understand my concerns.

If you have epilepsy and are thinking about becoming pregnant, this book will give you the basic facts that you will need in order to make appropriate decisions about preparing yourself for pregnancy, becoming pregnant, labor and delivery, and the early days after childbirth. Discuss the information in this book with your doctors because it should be interpreted in the light of your own particular circumstances. Keep in mind that knowledge about the interactions between epilepsy and pregnancy is always changing.

Epilepsy and seizures affect 2.5 million Americans of all ages, from babies to elders, at an estimated annual cost of $12.5 billion in direct and indirect costs. Ten percent of the American population will experience a seizure some time during their lifetime. Approximately 181,000 new cases of seizures and epilepsy occur each year. I developed epilepsy at the age of 5, following viral encephalitis.

It was very hard for me to accept my disorder. I was in denial for many years and felt sorry for myself. Finally, I joined a research group because I was desperate to find a "magic" drug that would help control my seizures. I met epileptics with brain damage and people who were so drugged they could not talk. I saw people who were having up to 60 seizures a day—some an hour and a half long!

Finally, I realized that I was lucky, because I was able to function and experience the joys of life. So I began to make an effort and eventually learned to cope with my disorder. During this time, I went to a bookstore for information, but found no more than five books on the shelf about epilepsy. All of them had been written by doctors, and only doctors could understand them. This compelled me to write my first book, *Epilepsy: You Are Not Alone.* I did research, interviewed 300 people with the disorder, and used my own experiences to help others cope with epilepsy and learn to live happier, healthier, and more productive lives. I conducted many seminars, became involved with the Epilepsy Foundation, appeared on television programs, wrote articles, and had articles written about me. For my efforts, the Epilepsy Foundation honored me with the Epilepsy Foundation of New Jersey Outstanding Volunteer Award, in June 2003.

Even though I had come to the realization that having epilepsy was not going to prevent me from being happy and productive, I still worried about what might happen if I tried to become a mother. I wanted to have my own children. I did not want to adopt, but I did not want to bring a baby into the world with Down syndrome or some other birth defect. I felt it would be selfish. There was a great deal to take into consideration.

After extensive research, consultations with my doctors, and long discussions with my husband, we came to the decision that we were going to have a baby. My doctors watched me closely, and I had a lot of tests and blood work. They started me on folic acid a couple of weeks before I became pregnant. I was nervous during my pregnancy and tried to do everything right. I ate nutritious food, steamed my vegetables, and always had a good night's sleep. I took my medicine on time and did everything the doctor told me to do. I had monthly blood tests. I had my EEGs and sonograms. And most important, I reported all my seizures to my neurologist so that he was able to adjust my medicine accordingly.

I was scared. I wasn't sure if the medicine I was taking for my seizures would cause birth defects. I was afraid the baby would be born with Down syndrome. Many issues crossed my mind, but I was determined to have a family of my own. When I looked up the percentage of birth defects in babies whose mothers have epilepsy compared to those who do not, I found there wasn't much difference.

I had a wonderful pregnancy with no complications. I was not tired until my 7th month. My doctor prescribed Trileptal and phenobarbital to prevent seizures. Trileptal is used frequently in Europe with pregnant women who have epilepsy. I actually had fewer seizures when I was pregnant than when I was not pregnant. I gave birth to Michael at 8¹/₂ months. He was healthy and had no birth defects.

I now have three healthy children: Michael, who is 5 years old; Alexis, who just turned 3; and Anthony, who is 7 months old. All my pregnancies were easy, and I had no complications, and no nausea. All three children were healthy, and the medicine I was taking to control the seizures did not affect them. The vast majority of women with epilepsy have uncomplicated pregnancies with normal deliveries and healthy children.

In the past, women with epilepsy have been discouraged from having children, and sometimes they were sterilized against their will to prevent pregnancy. When I was young, others told me there was a possibility that I might not be able to have children. Despite what others said, I knew deep down that when the time was right, I would focus on having a child.

After my third pregnancy, I decided to write a book for pregnant women with epilepsy. I had spoken with many women over the years who had epilepsy, many of whom were afraid to have children because of possible birth defects. They were afraid that the medication they were taking for epilepsy would have a negative effect on the baby. They were afraid they would have more frequent seizures or their seizures would become more severe.

These are common worries, but keep in mind that every person's seizure disorder is different. Some women have focal seizures; some have grand mal seizures; and each woman reacts differently to various medications. The seizures experienced by some women can be controlled with medication, and some cannot. Some seizures are derived from the left or right temporal part of the brain; some are from the frontal part; and some are derived from all parts of the brain.

Each woman's pregnancy is different, depending on the type of epilepsy she has, her past medical history, and the past medical history of her family. Women who have epilepsy and are considering pregnancy should first consult with their doctor to find out if it is a good idea to have children. According to scientific evidence, you *can* have healthy children even if you have epilepsy. Women with epilepsy can be great mothers.

Spiritually, I learned what my wants and needs are. I have also learned that I cannot let having epilepsy control my life. Yes, I have epilepsy, but life goes on! Epilepsy should not prevent you from enjoying life. People with epilepsy can work, care for children, go out with friends, play sports, and have meaningful relationships.

I am proud of whom I am, and I am determined to live a normal life. You cannot compare your life to someone else's. If you do, you are going to be unhappy. You need to love yourself and be satisfied with the life you lead. Change your life if you are not satisfied with it! There are plenty of people who take medicine and many individuals who do not drive for many other reasons.

We all have a special beauty within us—no one is perfect or has a life that is flawless. So do not be ashamed that you are epileptic. It is very easy to feel sorry for yourself, until you realize that some people have it much worse. Knowing that there are many other epileptics in this world also helps to make me feel better. We may have different seizures, but our feelings about living with epilepsy are all very similar.

I am committed to helping individuals with seizure disorders and developmental disabilities. I am also aware of the challenges and triumphs of helping individuals and their families who have disorders or disabilities. Still, I am determined to conquer any obstacles that get in my way, so that I can continue to help individuals who have a disorder to live healthy, happy, and productive lives.

Stacey Chillemi

EPILEPSY
AND PREGNANCY

Preconception Counseling

If you have epilepsy and you are planning to have a baby, make an appointment to see your neurologist or epileptologist (a physician who specializes in the treatment of epilepsy) for preconception counseling *before* trying to become pregnant. Many important issues need to be discussed and understood before you become pregnant, some of which you may be aware of, but many of which you may not be. Unfortunately, women often wait until they are already pregnant before calling their doctor.

Preconception counseling can have a major positive impact on the health of mothers and babies. This usually involves meeting with an epileptologist and other medical professionals who are experienced in both epilepsy and pregnancy. Preconception counseling usually consists of an assessment of the health of both potential parents, although a greater emphasis is usually placed on the woman with epilepsy. It may also involve some medical tests.

Women who take antiepileptic drugs (AEDs) to control their seizures need to understand that the medication can affect the baby. They also need to consider the possible effects of *not* taking medication: seizures during pregnancy can possibly harm the mother and her fetus. Preconception counseling can help women become fully educated about the interactions between epilepsy, AEDs, and pregnancy.

This is a good time to talk about any changes in your epilepsy treatment that might be necessary. The baby's main organs and skeleton develop during the first 4 months of pregnancy, a period during which AEDs may affect the fetus the most. This is one of the major reasons your epilepsy treatment should be evaluated before you get pregnant.

If a pregnant woman is having seizures, her AEDs may be kept at the lowest dose that allows for the best control of her seizures. Women who are likely to have seizures during pregnancy are also generally advised to keep taking their AEDs; however, your physician may recommend changes in the type of medication or the dose. *Do not change your AED dosage without consulting your doctor.*

If a woman has been free of seizures for 2 to 3 years, she may be able to stop taking her AEDs slowly, but there is always a chance that her seizures will recur. This needs to be cautiously and well thought out before a decision is made. Having seizures could affect the woman's everyday life, and she could also lose her driver's license.

There will be no opportunity for preconception counseling if an unplanned pregnancy occurs. In this case, you should continue to take your AEDs and see your epileptologist as soon as possible.

Birth Control

Birth control is important in preventing unplanned pregnancy. Understand your body and protect yourself from getting pregnant until you are ready to do so. Women who have epilepsy can use the following birth control methods:

❖ *Diaphragm:* The diaphragm is a shallow, dome-shaped cup with a flexible rim that fits securely in the vagina and covers the cervix. Diaphragms are used in conjunction with spermicidal creams.

❖ *Spermicidal vaginal cream:* Vaginal spermicides are chemical compounds that contain one ingredient that kills sperm, and another that provides a harmless base for the spermicidal agent.

❖ *Intrauterine device (IUD):* The IUD is a small, T-shaped, flexible device that is inserted into the uterine cavity by a doctor. IUDs can be inert, copper-releasing, or progestin-releasing. Copper-releasing IUDs interfere with the ability of sperm to pass through the uterine cavity and with the reproductive process before ova (eggs) reach the uterine cavity.

❖ *Condoms:* These are sheaths made of thin latex that are worn by the man during intercourse to prevent sperm from entering the uterine cavity.

❖ *Rhythm method:* Using this method of birth control, intercourse is avoided when the woman is fertile, the period during which an egg, or eggs, is released from the ovaries (ovulation).

❖ *Hormonal birth control:* This type of birth control is often prescribed by a doctor in the form of birth control pills (oral contraceptives), which contain hormones that prevent ovulation. They are taken daily to prevent pregnancy. Combination birth control pills containing synthetic estrogen and progesterone are the most commonly prescribed. Hormones may also be administered via hormonal implants or hormone injections.

Hormonal contraception is the most dependable method for most women, but it is not 100% successful (no birth control method is), especially for women who have epilepsy. There is always a slim chance of an unwanted pregnancy, even with the correct usage of contraceptives: 0.7 pregnancies occur per 100 women-years of birth control coverage in women taking birth control pills consistently.

There can be interactions between the estrogen and progesterone contained in birth control pills or devices and some of the medications used to control seizures. Some AEDs increase the breakdown of contraceptive hormones in the body, making them less effective in preventing pregnancy. The AEDs that have this effect are often called liver-enzyme-inducing medications, because the liver is the organ that breaks down hormones. These AEDs include the following:

Brand Name	Generic Name
Dilantin	phenytoin
Lamictal	lamotrigine
Mysoline	primidone
n/a	phenobarbital
Tegretol	carbamazepine
Topamax	topiramate
Trileptal	oxcarbazepine

The following AEDs do *not* increase the breakdown of hormones, and do *not* interfere with the effectiveness of hormonal birth control. They may even increase hormonal levels, necessitating a change in the dose of hormonal birth control.

Brand Name	Generic Name
Depakote	valproic acid
Felbatol	felbamate
Gabitril	tiagabine
Keppra	levetiracetam
Neurontin	gabapentin

There are also other concerns about women with epilepsy using birth control pills. The low-dose, combined oral contraceptive pill has a relatively small amount of estrogen (less than 35 mcg). This is not enough to prevent pregnancy in women with epilepsy who take enzyme-inducing AEDs. They may need birth control pills with a higher dose of estrogen, and even then, there is a risk of unexpected pregnancy. If you are taking an AED that increases the breakdown of the hormones in the pills, it is a good idea to use another birth control method, such as a diaphragm, spermicidal cream, or condoms, in addition to birth control pills.

Hormonal implants that are placed under the skin, such as Norplant, may not supply efficient birth control protection if you are taking certain epilepsy medications. The medications that cause the most frequent problems with Norplant are the same liver-enzyme-inducing AEDs listed above.

Depo-Provera is a hormonal injection used for birth control. These injections may be needed more frequently by women with epilepsy who are taking the medications listed previously.

Warning signs that hormonal birth control is not working properly may include breakthrough bleeding, which is bleeding at any time other than when normally expected. Note that hormonal contraception can also fail without breakthrough bleeding. If bleeding occurs, ask your doctor to help you select an additional form of contraception, such as the diaphragm, spermicidal vaginal cream, or condoms.

Having irregular periods can make hormonal birth control and the rhythm method less reliable. Typically, irregular menstrual cycles mean that the hormones are unstable in some way. It is important to tell your obstetrician and your neurologist or epileptologist if your periods are irregular, so she or he can help you choose the best method of contraception. It may also be necessary to talk with an endocrinologist (a physician who specializes in diagnosing and treating hormonal problems).

Scientific research does not indicate a consistent change in the number of seizures that occur when women with epilepsy use hormonal birth control, but individual reports indicate that changes are possible. Some women have reported more seizures, others fewer. Contact your physician if you notice a change in your seizure pattern when you use hormonal birth control.

Issues to Discuss and Questions to Ask

The following topics should be discussed during preconception counseling:

❖ Weight: The time to reach your appropriate weight is *before* you decide to have a baby. Obesity may put your pregnancy in a high-risk category. Women who are underweight sometimes ovulate irregularly, or they do not ovulate at all, making it difficult to get pregnant.

❖ Diet: A healthy diet is necessary before, during, and after pregnancy.

❖ Folic acid: This vitamin is essential in preventing fetal malformations, such as neural tube defects and spina bifida, and fetal cardiac problems. This protection applies to the very early stages of pregnancy, so it is vital to start folic acid supplementation at least 1 to 2 months before you conceive.

❖ Home and workspace environment: Remove anything that might be harmful, such as lead paint, asbestos, and toxic chemicals. Cat litter boxes should be handled carefully or eliminated in order to prevent toxoplasmosis, which can be transmitted via cat feces to humans. This infection can damage the human central nervous system, especially that of infants.

❖ Smoking and alcohol: Do not smoke if you are considering becoming pregnant; ask your doctor for help with quitting. This goes for your partner, too. If you drink alcohol, stop as soon as you start trying to conceive.

❖ Risk factors: Discuss the risk factors for major malformations, minor anomalies, and developmental disturbances in the fetus or infant, taking into account family history, type and severity of epilepsy, and/or intrauterine AED exposure.

❖ Pregnancy complications: Discuss the risk factors for pregnancy complications, such as bleeding, toxemia, and prematurity that may result from AED therapy.

❖ Seizure control and timing of pregnancy: Let your doctor know if you have had frequent major seizures during the year preceding the time you are trying to conceive.

❖ Medications: As noted above, women with epilepsy who are planning to have children should discuss their AEDs thoroughly with their doctors before conceiving, and make any necessary adjustments in AED or dosage.

❖ German measles: Request a blood test for German measles if you do not know whether you have had it in the past or been vaccinated against it. German measles during pregnancy can harm the baby. If necessary, get vaccinated before you get pregnant.

❖ Sexually transmitted diseases: STDs, such as gonorrhea, syphilis, chlamydia, and AIDS, can make it difficult to get pregnant. They can also harm the mother and the baby. STDs should be diagnosed and treated before pregnancy.

Ask your epileptologist the following and any similar questions that you may have:

❖ Is there a possibility my child will have epilepsy? Can it be inherited?

❖ Can my medication be reduced or are there safer medications that I can take while pregnant, especially during the first 4 months?

❖ What are my options for AED withdrawal? (Any drug withdrawal should be completed at least 6 months before planned conception, because the risk of seizure recurrence after AED withdrawal is the greatest during the first 6 months.)

❖ Can my epilepsy be controlled with just one medication?

❖ How will my AEDs affect the baby and me while I am pregnant?

❖ Can anything be done to decrease the chance of birth defects?

❖ Will having a baby affect my need for AEDs or the dose?

❖ Will morning sickness affect my AEDs?

❖ Will my seizures be different during pregnancy?

❖ Do I need any vaccinations?

Your epileptologist, obstetrician, and other health care professionals can help prevent many possible problems for you and your baby, so it is best to see them for preconception counseling before you get pregnant, while you are pregnant, and after the baby is born.

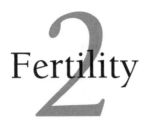

Fertility

Many people think getting pregnant is easy, but a woman having regular unprotected intercourse has, on average, only a 20% to 25% chance each month of getting pregnant. Surprisingly, one half of all couples try for more than 6 months before the woman conceives.

The fertility rate of women with epilepsy is 25% to 33% less than average, meaning women with epilepsy have fewer children. Women with epilepsy are less likely to marry and may choose not to have children. Societal pressure may also play a role in making the decision to have children. Women with epilepsy have a higher rate of menstrual irregularities, polycystic ovary syndrome, and reproductive endocrine disorders. Any of these factors may decrease the chances of conceiving.

Fertility problems related to epilepsy can be treated. Women with epilepsy who need fertility treatment—often for reasons unrelated to their epilepsy—should have their epilepsy medications withdrawn or adjusted before they start fertility treatment. The medications that are given to increase egg production may also increase seizures. Note that seizures may reoccur if AEDs are withdrawn, even if seizures have been controlled. This predisposition usually settles very quickly.

Conception is sometimes more difficult for women with epilepsy, who may have anovulatory cycles (cycles in which no egg is released). They are more likely to have irregular periods, making it difficult to calculate the time of ovulation. This is partially the result of epilepsy, which can disturb the fragile balance of the hormones released in the brain that control the menstrual cycle. It may also result from the effect of seizure control medication on the ovaries.

Stacey Chillemi's Experience

I calculated ovulation using the rhythm method. First, I would mark the calendar on the day I menstruated; then I counted 14 days ahead and marked that day on the calendar with a circle. Next, I marked an

X 4 days before the circle and another X 4 days after the circle. In this way, I determined that I was fertile during the week between the two Xs. I would watch carefully for a stringy discharge when I urinated during this period of time, which I knew meant I was ovulating. I used this method each time I tried to conceive, and I got pregnant each time on the first try. I also used this method when I did not want to conceive, by avoiding intercourse during the time I was fertile. I never had an unplanned pregnancy.

Many women with epilepsy have polycystic ovary syndrome, a condition characterized by irregular ovulation and menses. The ovaries of women with this condition fail to release an egg at a regular time each month, making conception difficult. The infertility caused by this syndrome is treatable. Polycystic ovary syndrome may be more common in women with epilepsy, and there is some evidence that one particular medication that is used to control seizures (sodium valproate) may also bring on this syndrome. If this is true—and not all experts agree—this effect may be reversible. It is worth noting that many doctors warn women who stop taking sodium valproate that they may get pregnant easily, and that they should use contraception if they do not wish to become immediately pregnant. The policy of some doctors is to screen all adolescent girls with epilepsy—as well as women seeking preconception counseling—for the presence of polycystic ovaries and the associated hormonal changes, and advise them accordingly.

The Menstrual Cycle

The hypothalamic–pituitary axis—the part of the brain that controls all of the endocrine systems in the body—controls the female reproductive cycle, and disruption of this axis is associated with anovulatory cycles in women with epilepsy. Seizures may change how the hypothalamus secretes gonadotropin hormone. The change in the normal cycle of gonadotropin hormone release will in turn affect how pituitary hormone release occurs. It is the pituitary hormone release in cyclical fashion that controls the ovarian release of hormones and the menstrual cycle.

Seizure discharges in the brain disturb the hormone cycle control from the hypothalamus, and in turn, the pituitary, producing an epileptic-discharge-induced rise in the hormone LH, and a subsequent fall in LH after the discharge has stopped. (LH, or luteinizing hormone, helps regulate the menstrual cycle in women and causes ovulation to occur.) Different types of epilepsy may affect how LH is released, with an increase in the bursts of LH secretion in patients with generalized epilepsies, and a decrease in the bursts of LH release in those with temporal lobe epilepsy. Such disturbances in LH release in either direction may cause a woman to fail to ovulate and may therefore impair fertility.

Some antiepileptic drugs may stimulate an enzyme system in the liver so that it gets rid of circulating fertility-related hormones more quickly. The names of some of these hormones are estradiol, adrenal androgen, gonadal androgen, and sex-hormone-binding globulin (a substance that binds other hormones). Only a free hormone has biologically significant activity. When part of the circulating hormone is bound to another protein, it loses its biological activity. Therefore, when there is an increase in protein binding, there is a decrease in active hormone effect. Valproate (VPA) decreases the activity of the liver enzyme system that gets rid of hormones, producing an increase in androgen from the ovaries and from the endocrine glands lying on top of the kidneys (the adrenal glands). Gapapentin and lamotrigine are antiepileptic medications that do not have an effect on this system. Women receiving these medications to control seizures show no difference in gonadal steroids when compared with non-epileptic controls.

The menstrual cycle is a well-regulated cycle that can be susceptible to a number of stressors, such as physical or emotional stress. A normal cycle length is 23 to 35 days, and cycle-to-cycle variability should not exceed 5 days. One third of women with epilepsy have abnormal cycle lengths, compared with 8% of women without epilepsy. Women with epilepsy also bleed more frequently during their midcycle and have metrorrhagia (irregular intervals and excessive flow and duration). In addition, anovulatory cycles have been described in more than 30% of women with epilepsy. The clinical manifestations of anovulation include amenorrhea (absence of menses), irregular menses, and hirsutism (excess hairiness). The serious consequences of chronic anovulation are infertility and a greater risk for developing carcinoma of the endometrium and perhaps the breast.

Polycystic ovary syndrome (PCOS) is a gynecologic condition that affects 7% to 10% of women of reproductive age. Obesity, acne, hirsutism, elevated androgens, elevated LH/FSH ratio, abnormal lipid profile, chronic anovulation, and polycystic ovaries characterize PCOS. Not all of these features need be present. The required features are hyperandrogenism and frequent anovulatory cycles. An abnormality in the insulin receptor, causing insulin resistance, is the basis for PCOS. Long-term consequences of PCOS include infertility, dyslipidemia, glucose intolerance and diabetes, and endometrial cancer.

Approximately 30% of women with epilepsy have polycystic-appearing ovaries, compared with 15% of reproductive-aged women. Studies suggest that VPA is particularly associated with polycystic ovaries, hyperandrogenism, hyperinsulinemia, and obesity. Up to 60% of women with epilepsy who are receiving VPA have polycystic-appearing ovaries, compared with 25% to 30% of women with epilepsy receiving other antiepileptic medications. In one study, the prevalence was highest in women receiving VPA prior to age 20.

The signs and symptoms associated with VPA use appear to be reversible. In one study, 16 women taking VPA with polycystic-appearing ovaries, hyperandrogenism, and hyperinsulinemia were changed to lamotrigine. Polycystic-appearing ovaries resolved within 1 year in most of these women. Testosterone and insulin became normal within several months. Another study also found an association between current or recent use of VPA for epilepsy and anovulatory cycles and polycystic ovaries. Therefore, the reproductive and metabolic effects of VPA appear to be reversible for women with epilepsy.

Sexual dysfunction affects 30% to 40% of people with epilepsy. This may appear in women as diminished sexual interest and desire, and a disorder of sexual arousal that includes dyspareunia (chronic pelvic pain in the lower abdomen and pelvis that is not related to menstruation), vaginismus (painful, involuntary contractions of the vaginal muscles), and lack of lubrication. Antiepileptic medications may contribute to sexual dysfunction by direct cortical effects, or secondarily through alterations in the hormone effects on sexual behavior. Clinicians must be alert to signs of reproductive dysfunction in women with epilepsy receiving antiepileptic medications. Keeping a diary of the length of the menstrual cycle and timing and duration of menstrual flow is the most sensitive indicator for anovulatory cycles. Intermittent checking of ovulation with over-the-counter ovulation kits done over a consecutive 3-month period can be used to determine whether or not ovulation is occurring. Women with menstrual dysfunction should be referred for gynecologic evaluation and care.

Risks of Pregnancy

Risks to the Woman

Many women with epilepsy are worried about possible risks in becoming pregnant. Women with epilepsy who become pregnant do have a higher risk for complications than women who do not have epilepsy. This includes the possibility of having more frequent seizures, which can cause pregnant women to become sleepy or fall, possibly causing serious injury. Other women experience a *decrease* in the frequency of their seizures when they are pregnant.

Most women do not see any change in the frequency of their seizures when they are pregnant. Increased seizures are usually seen in women who do not take their AEDs as the doctor prescribes. Epilepsy may also occur for the first time in pregnancy.

The body processes AEDs differently during pregnancy. This can lead to medication levels that are too high (which can cause side effects) or too low (which can cause more seizures). Blood levels of medication usually become lower with the weight gain of pregnancy, and your neurologist will probably have to increase your dosage to limit unnecessary seizures. It is important to control seizures during pregnancy because it is safer for the baby and the mother. As stated previously, pregnant women who have epilepsy should not stop taking their AEDs without permission from their doctor. Each woman who has epilepsy will react differently to pregnancy and childbirth, and your doctor will discuss any possible risks, and monitor you and your fetus closely.

It can be useful for the medical team that is assisting with the birth to be aware of your medical history as it relates to your epilepsy disorder, such as medication and seizure types.

Tonic-clonic seizures (convulsions with muscular rigidity) can cause miscarriage or injury to the baby in rare circumstances. Only 1% to 2% of women with uncontrolled epilepsy will have a tonic-clonic seizure in labor; 1% to 2% will have some type of seizure in the 24 hours after birth. Medication can be used to control seizures in the event one occurs during labor.

Pregnant women with epilepsy who want to have a home birth need to consider the complications that could arise if a seizure occurs during labor. Water births also need to be carefully considered, because consciousness may be impaired during seizures. A water birth can be performed at home or at a birthing center. The warm water relaxes the mother's back and pelvic muscles, and takes the weight of the baby off the mother's back and hips. Relaxation, combined with the buoyancy of water, helps the baby descend through the birth canal. A water birth can provide a relaxing transition for the baby from the womb into the world.

Potential obstetrical complications that are seen more frequently in women with epilepsy include vaginal bleeding, anemia, and hyperemesis gravidarum (HG), a rare disorder characterized by severe and persistent nausea and vomiting during pregnancy that may necessitate hospitalization. As a result of frequent nausea and vomiting, affected women experience dehydration, vitamin and mineral deficit, and the loss of greater than 5% of their original body weight. Difficulties during labor and delivery include premature labor, failure to progress, and an increased rate of cesarean section, which may become necessary to protect the well-being of the mother or baby.

Approximately 1 million women of childbearing age in the United States have epilepsy. Complications may arise during conception and pregnancy that involve the choice of AED, when to take the medication, and how to control seizures. These complications have social as well as medical ramifications for pregnant women and their families. During pregnancy, factors such as the choice of AEDs for seizure control, hormonal changes, and vitamin deficiencies can have some bearing on seizure patterns, even for women who have had excellent seizure control before becoming pregnant. These complications, combined with genetic factors, can also lead to a greater risk for major and minor birth defects for babies born to women with epilepsy. Although this risk is not usually significant enough for neurologists and epileptologists to advise their patients against pregnancy, health care specialists support a careful and cautious pregnancy for all women who have, or have had, epilepsy.

As stated earlier, the number of seizures remains unchanged during pregnancy for most women. However, about 20% will experience an increase in seizures during pregnancy. Some women experience seizures *only* during birth. The physiologic changes that may play a role in the increased incidence of seizures for some women include changes in hormone production, metabolism, stress, and alteration in sleeping patterns.

The hormones estrogen and progesterone increase naturally and steadily during normal pregnancy. Estrogen has been shown to be epileptogenic (increasing seizure activity), and progesterone is thought to have an anti-seizure effect. Fluctuations in the levels of these hormones can make it more difficult for mothers who are epileptic to predict and control their seizures.

Generally, sleep deprivation influences seizure frequency for those who have epilepsy. A significant increase in seizure occurrence may result during pregnancy when sleep patterns change. Stress, and the associated changes in eating and sleeping habits, may also contribute to an increase in seizures for some women.

In most cases, the level of AEDs in the blood decreases during pregnancy despite adherence to the proper dosage. For many women, this does not result in an increase in seizures. In the majority of instances in which seizures increase, the levels of AEDs in the blood are found to be lower than the recommended therapeutic range. It is therefore very important to monitor medication levels closely during pregnancy.

Risks to the Baby

One of your first questions when considering whether to have a baby may be, Is there any risk of birth defects or problems after birth?

More than 90% of women with epilepsy have normal, healthy babies, but there are some risks, including vaginal bleeding during pregnancy, premature birth, and delays in development and growth of the baby, as well as the possibility of birth defects caused by AEDs. Pregnant women who do not take their medication, however, may experience even greater risks to themselves and their babies. Uncontrolled seizures, particularly generalized tonic-clonic episodes, are dangerous during pregnancy. Maternal seizures can cause miscarriage, trauma related to falls, fetal hypoxia (lack of oxygen to the baby), and acidosis (an increase in the acidity of body fluids). Status epilepticus (a seizure lasting more than 30 minutes) carries a high mortality rate for mother and fetus, and generalized seizures occurring during labor can result in fetal bradycardia (slowing of the heartbeat).

Major malformations are defined as defects of medical, surgical, or cosmetic importance. These problems can seriously affect a child's life, and occur in 2% to 3% of all live births. The incidence is estimated to be 4% to 8% for women with epilepsy who are taking one AED, and possibly greater for women taking more than one AED. The types of major malformations that occur most often in children of women with epilepsy are facial clefts, cardiac abnormalities, and neural tube (spine and brain) defects.

Babies born to mothers with epilepsy have a higher risk of being stillborn, which is defined as the delivery of a nonliving baby after the 20th week of pregnancy. (Loss of a fetus before the 20th week of pregnancy is considered a miscarriage.)

As discussed in chapter 1, folic acid supplementation (at a minimum dose of 0.4 mg daily) is especially important prior to conception and during pregnancy for women with epilepsy in order to lower the risk of neural tube defects in the offspring.

In general, AED polypharmacy and higher blood levels of AEDs are associated with the increased incidence of birth defects in infants born to women with epilepsy. A single AED at the lowest possible dose for efficacy is recommended whenever possible.

The numbers of minor physical defects in infants born to women with epilepsy is approximately 15%. Possible defects include the following:

❖ *Hypertelorism*—an abnormally increased distance between two structures.

❖ *Epicanthic fold*—a fold of skin that partly covers the inner corner of the eyes, which is present in some chromosome abnormalities (Down syndrome, for example).

❖ *Shallow philtrum*—shallowness in the vertical groove above the middle of the upper lip.

❖ *Distal digital hypoplasia*—incomplete development of the last joint of the fingers. The joint is a smaller size and often has a smaller fingernail.

❖ *Simian crease*—a single line across the middle of the palm of the hand, as is seen in monkeys and apes, as opposed to the two or three broken lines seen in humans.

Although the incidence of the defects previously listed is reported to be 2 to 3 times greater in women with epilepsy, they may be present in infants whose mothers used other types of medication or drank alcohol excessively during pregnancy. Many of these minor physical defects appear to be idiopathic (without a clear cause) in nature, and do not cause any serious problems. They are primarily of cosmetic concern.

Babies born to women with epilepsy may have a slightly greater risk of developing seizures as they get older. The causes of most types of seizure disorders are varied, and so the occurrence of epilepsy in children born to epileptic parents varies. Children whose mothers have epilepsy have about a 3% chance of inheriting it. If only the father is affected by epilepsy, the risk is the same as it is for anyone in the general public. The risk rises to approximately 5% if both parents have epilepsy.

As noted previously, research has determined that some AEDs are categorized as high risk, and should be avoided, withdrawn, or substituted before conception, if necessary. Some medications are medium risk, and should be withdrawn or substituted if possible, particularly if they are taken in combination with another drug. Medium-risk medications taken in a low dose—with no other medications and with the addition of folic acid—are reasonably safe. Some AEDs are considered low risk. According to the available research, these medications have no more risk than the risk that is usually associated with epilepsy itself (this view is largely based on experiments with animals).

Categories of AEDs

HIGH-RISK MEDICATIONS

Brand Name	Generic Name
Depakote	valproic acid
Dilantin	phenytoin
n/a	phenobarbital
Mysoline	primidone

MEDIUM-RISK MEDICATIONS

Brand Name	Generic Name
Frisium	clobozam
Klonopin	clonazepam
Sabrin	vigabatrin
Tegretol	carbamazepine
Topamax	topirimate
Trileptol	oxcarbazepine
Zarontin	ethosuximide

Low-Risk Medication

Brand Name	Generic Name
Lamictal	lamotrigine
Neurontin	gabapentin
Gabitril	tiagabine
Keppra	levetiracetam

Of the high-risk medications, only valproate is likely to be taken by women of childbearing age. Doctors might try to remove valproate if there is a family or previous history of spina bifida (a neural tube birth defect in which the bones of the spine do not form properly around the spinal cord). The present medical policy is to avoid using this drug in women of childbearing potential unless it is the only drug that will help them. Valproate is often, but not always, withdrawn, or lamotrigine is substituted. Withdrawal or substitution is a long, slow process, however. If it is impossible to completely withdraw from valproate, physicians often reduce the dose as much as possible, and suggest it be taken 3 to 4 times a day. The hope is that spreading out the dose in this way will reduce the risk of seizures.

It is important to remember that even with a high-risk medication, most babies born to mothers with epilepsy are fine. Studies have focused on abnormality at birth, but there are some data that show a minority of the babies born to mothers taking AEDs are physically small, with small heads and delayed development. They catch up in size eventually, but there is research suggesting that some of these babies may have specific learning problems later on. This may be particularly likely with mothers taking sodium valproate for epilepsy. Further research is urgently needed to clarify the extent of this problem. As babies are developing, some—not all—tend to be less likely to learn quickly. The development of language skills may be slower. This condition affects 2% to 6% of births and differs from retardation in that children with developmental delay sometimes are not permanently impaired, although it is uncertain how many of them catch up.

The most dangerous period for problems caused by AEDs seems to be approximately the first 56 days of pregnancy, when the main organs and skeleton are developing. The risk after 4 months of pregnancy is thought to be very low. As discussed in chapter 1, it is important to discuss your AEDs with your doctor and to start taking folic acid before trying to get pregnant, because the most vulnerable period starts before you know you are pregnant, particularly if you have an irregular cycle. Women who get pregnant easily may be temporarily weaned from their epilepsy medication before conception and then resume it after they are about 4 months pregnant, although this can be risky.

Stacey Chillemi's Experience

When I was pregnant with my third child, my neurologist was in the process of weaning me off one of my AEDs and putting me on another AED so that my seizures could be controlled later. The new medication didn't agree with me during pregnancy, and the seizures increased. I was only a few weeks pregnant, so my neurologist weaned me off the new AED and put me on the same AED at the same dosage that I had been on during my previous pregnancies. As a result, my seizures decreased, and I had fewer seizures during my pregnancy than before.

Pregnancy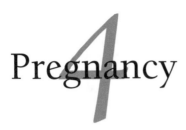

Women with epilepsy have a 90% chance of having a healthy, normal baby. The chance that children of parents with epilepsy will also develop the disorder depends on the type of epilepsy the parents have and whether it is a hereditary form of the disorder. There are two main factors in the cause of epilepsy. One is whether the person has had an injury to the brain, such as from an accident or an infection. The other factor is the *seizure threshold*.

The seizure threshold is a person's level of resistance to seizures. Everyone has a seizure threshold, and anyone can have a seizure under certain conditions. People with a low seizure threshold may suddenly start having seizures. People with a high threshold are less likely to start having seizures unless something specific happens, such as an injury to the brain.

The seizure threshold is part of the genetic makeup that is passed on from parent to child. There may be several people with epilepsy in some families; in others, there may be only one. The chance of a child's developing epilepsy depends on the seizure threshold of both parents (if they have epilepsy).

Sometimes epilepsy is part of an inherited medical condition. This is rare, but includes neurofibromatosis and tuberous sclerosis. Neurofibromatosis is a familial condition producing multiple soft tumors that may appear in the nervous system, muscles, bone, and skin along with pigmented areas. Tuberous sclerosis is a rare genetic multisystem disorder that is typically obvious shortly after birth. The disorder may be characterized by episodes of uncontrolled electrical activity in the brain (seizures); mental retardation; distinctive skin abnormalities (lesions); and benign (noncancerous), tumorlike nodules (hamartomas) of the brain, certain regions of the eyes (retinas), the heart, the kidneys, the lungs, or other tissues or organs.

Genes play a part in the development of epilepsy, but their importance varies. Every situation is different, and women with epilepsy are advised to consult a geneticist (a doctor who specializes in genetics). The geneticist can help determine the chances of the baby's developing a specific type of epilepsy. Tests performed by the doctor (amniocentesis and ultrasound) can help determine that the baby is developing normally.

Because AEDs can slightly increase the risk for birth defects, most doctors ask women with epilepsy to tell them at least 3 months in advance if they plan to conceive so their AEDs can be adjusted, if necessary, and folic acid and multivitamins can be prescribed. If you become pregnant before consulting your doctor, however, you should continue taking your medications as prescribed. Once you tell your doctor you are pregnant, the doctor will probably prescribe blood tests. The test results, the medications you are taking, and the number of seizures you may be having will help determine the amount of medication you should take on a daily basis.

Each year about 20,000 women with epilepsy become pregnant. Over the years, that number has increased because of increased marriage rates, and because society has accepted the fact that men and women with epilepsy can be great parents and do just as well as anyone else. During that time, the epilepsy community has made tremendous progress through research for pregnant women. New tests and procedures have made it possible to watch the development of the fetus and detect any abnormalities before birth.

During your pregnancy, the number of seizures you have may change. For pregnant women with preexisting epilepsy, approximately 35% experience more frequent seizures, 55% have no change in the frequency of seizures, and approximately 10% have fewer seizures during pregnancy.

The reasons women may experience changes in the number of seizures include:

- ❖ Changes in sex hormones
- ❖ Changes in AED metabolism, volume, or distribution
- ❖ Changes in renal clearance (the rate at which the kidneys are able to clear the plasma of a substance) or protein binding
- ❖ Changes in sleep schedules
- ❖ Irregularity in taking medication

The concentration of AEDs may change during pregnancy. A number of physiologic changes during pregnancy can alter the effect of AEDs, including the following:

- ❖ Changes in stomach and intestinal absorption of AEDs
- ❖ Decreased gastric tone (which determines the sensitivity of the stomach to distention)

❖ Motility (the movement of foods in the gastrointestinal system)

❖ Increase in renal clearance

Albumin, a major protein in plasma, is a volume expander. As it expands, it helps to keep the blood from leaking out of the blood vessels. Fluid may collect in the ankles, lungs, or abdomen when albumin levels drop. Albumin is vital for tissue development and healing. It is also needed for protein binding, as the carrier proteins that carry substances around the blood, including antiepileptic drugs.

One part of antiepileptic drugs—the biologically active part—occurs free (unbound) in the blood. Because there is an increase in the free part of AEDs when both albumin levels and protein binding decline, it is necessary to follow the nonprotein-bound drug concentration (the free level) of AEDS, especially for AEDS that are highly protein-bound, such as carbamazepine, phenytoin, and valproic acid. The unbound or free portion of antiepileptic drugs in some cases may provide more accurate clinical information to your physician.

Controlling seizures during pregnancy is extremely important, because women with epilepsy are at greater risk for miscarriage. The reasons for miscarriage are not completely understood, but they are probably related more to maternal seizures than to the fetus's being exposed to AEDs. This is supported by the finding of fetal heart rate decelerations during maternal seizures.

The older medications that control seizures, such as the benzodiazepines, phenytoin, carbamazepine, phenobarbital, and valproic acid, are teratogenic, meaning they can cause birth defects if a woman gets pregnant while she is taking them. Minor malformations present at birth, including facial dysmorphism (abnormal shape of the face) and digital anomalies (minor abnormalities in the developmental and shape of the fingers), occur in 6% to 20% of infants exposed to AEDs in utero. This is approximately a twofold increase over the general population. These defects are typically slight and are often outgrown. The most common birth defects are cleft lip and palate. Cleft palate is a non-life-threatening birth defect in which there is a split in the roof of the mouth.

Cardiac defects and urogenital defects (structural abnormalities of the kidney and sexual organ system) occur in 4% to 6% of babies born to mothers with epilepsy who are taking the older types of AEDs (such as phenobarbital), compared with 2% to 4% of the general population. Neural tube defects such as spinal bifida and anencephaly (absence of the brain and spinal cord) occur in 0.5% to 1% of infants exposed to carbamazepine, and 1% to 2% of infants exposed to valproic acid during the first trimester. The risk of birth defects is highest in fetuses exposed to multiple medications and in those exposed to higher dosages. A study confirmed these observations, finding an increased number of major birth defects, growth retardation, microcephaly (abnormal smallness of the head), and hypoplasia (incomplete development) of the midface or fingers in children born to mothers taking two or more of the older AEDs.

Since 1993, a number of new medications for epilepsy have been available for usage. The U.S. National Pregnancy Registry has little information regarding the teratogenicity of the newer medications for epilepsy. All of these are listed by the Food and Drug Administration as Use-in-Pregnancy Risk Category C medications—meaning the risks are not known and therefore cannot be ruled out. Registries have been established to gather data about fetal outcome after exposure to the newer AEDs.

In the United States, the Antiepileptic Drug Registry can be reached by telephone (1-888-233-2334) or at the registry's Web site (www.aed pregnancyregistry.org). Pregnant women with epilepsy can enroll in this registry if they want to participate in studies. Participation in these studies will help doctors understand epilepsy and pregnancy and enable them to find new ways to help women with epilepsy. The main goal of the studies is to help future mothers have a safe pregnancy with as few seizures as possible.

Although the data are limited, there are increasing concerns that exposure to AEDs in utero may have long-lasting, unfavorable neurodevelopmental or neurocognitive effects. A retrospective study found that children exposed in utero to valproic acid in monotherapy (single-drug therapy) or polytherapy (multiple-drug therapy) were more likely to require special educational resources. Prospective studies are underway to describe better the neurodevelopmental risks to the developing brain from exposure to AEDs.

Folic acid deficiency is a possible cause of teratogenicity for phenytoin, carbamazepine, phenobarbital, and valproic acid. Unfortunately, there are no definitive studies on the effect of folic acid supplementation in women with epilepsy, and several studies report inconsistent results. For example, one study associated lower serum levels of folic acid with a higher risk of defects in children of mothers taking folic acid during their pregnancy. Another reported a decrease in children who were born with major malformations when their mothers took folic acid during pregnancy. Still others reported no decrease in the risk of non-neural-tube defects, such as cleft lip and palate and cardiovascular and urinary tract malformations for the babies born of mothers who took folic acid during pregnancy. There was a report of one baby who was born with a neural tube defect to a mother who took 2,000 mg of valproic acid per day and folic acid.

Although there has been insufficient research, many medical societies, including the American Academy of Neurology, the American College of Obstetric and Gynecologic Physicians, and the Canadian Society of Medical Geneticists, suggest that all women of childbearing age who take medicine to control seizures should also take folic acid at 0.4–5.0 mg per day. The U.S. Centers for Disease Control also recommends that all women of childbearing age receive routine supplementation of folic acid of at least 0.4 mg per day.

The most popular way to control seizures during pregnancy is monotherapy at the lowest effective dosage, whenever possible. The best AED to take while you are pregnant is the one that controls *your* seizures and is well tolerated. At the time of this writing, there is not enough information to distinguish any particular seizure medication that is the safest during pregnancy. It would be wonderful to have just one medication that could control all seizures for every person who has epilepsy. Unfortunately, this is not likely to happen soon. Until then, pregnant women with epilepsy should work with their neurologists to find the best alternatives.

Pregnant women with epilepsy will need to see a neurologist or epileptologist and obstetrician more often than pregnant women who do not have epilepsy. These health care professionals monitor pregnancy closely in order to ensure the best outcome for mothers and their babies.

Prenatal Testing

Urine and blood tests are given throughout pregnancy, as is routine blood pressure screening. Other tests, listed below, may be offered if the pregnant woman's age or other factors indicate that she or her baby are at higher risk for certain conditions or diseases.

ULTRASOUND

Ultrasound is a method of imaging the fetus and the female pelvic organs during pregnancy.

Procedure

The ultrasound device sends out high-frequency sound waves that bounce off body structures to create a picture.

Risks

The risks of ultrasound are minimal.

Diagnosis

Some doctors perform a scan at around 13 or 14 weeks of pregnancy to screen for developmental abnormalities in the fetus. The total number of scans will vary, depending on whether a previous scan or blood tests have detected abnormalities that require follow-up evaluation. Ultrasound scans may be performed during the first trimester to confirm a normal intrauterine pregnancy, assess fetal age, assess fetal heart activity, determine the presence of multiple pregnancies, and identify abnormalities of the placenta, uterus, or other pelvic structures.

Scans may also be obtained during the second and third trimesters to assess fetal age, growth, position, and sometimes gender; identify congenital malformations of the face, brain, spinal column, heart and other internal organs, and the limbs; exclude multiple pregnancies; and evaluate the placenta, amniotic fluid, and remaining structures of the pelvis.

CHORIONIC VILLUS SAMPLING (CVS)

This test can detect genetic abnormalities earlier than amniocentesis can, and may be performed when you are 8 to 12 weeks pregnant.

Procedure

The chorionic villi are small cylindrical extensions on the placenta that have the same genetic makeup as the fetus. Using ultrasound as a guide, a fine tube is passed through the cervix, or sometimes through the abdomen, to remove a sample of chorionic tissue.

Risks

The risks include infection, maternal bleeding, miscarriage, and birth defects.

Diagnosis

CVS can detect a number of genetic problems in the fetus, but not all of them. If a genetic problem is identified, the parents must then face a decision about what action they will take, including whether to terminate the pregnancy.

NUCHAL SCAN

A nuchal scan test can be performed at 10 weeks to screen for Down syndrome (a type of chromosomal defect that causes mental retardation).

Procedure

The depth of the dark, fluid-filled space behind the baby's neck is measured using an ultrasound scanner. The deeper this space is, the greater the risk of Down syndrome.

Risks

The risks of the nuchal scan test are minimal. This test is not diagnostic and only predicts risk, so it may cause unnecessary concern.

Diagnosis

An approximation of the risk of Down syndrome can be made. This test is only for Down syndrome.

AMNIOCENTESIS

Amniocentesis may be performed to test for birth defects, including Down syndrome.

Procedure

Amniocentesis is performed by inserting a hollow needle through the abdominal wall into the uterus, using ultrasound as a guide, and withdrawing a small amount of fluid from the sac surrounding the fetus.

Risks

There are serious risks to consider, including miscarriage, although the risks are generally lower than they are with CVS.

Diagnosis

Normal results will be reassuring, but no test can guarantee a healthy baby. If the results show an abnormality, the parents may face the difficult decision of whether to continue the pregnancy.

BLOOD TESTS

Blood tests can be performed at about 14 weeks to identify certain problems with the fetus.

Procedure

A sample of blood is taken from the mother and analyzed for the levels of alpha-fetoprotein (AFP) and human chorionic gonadotropin (HCG).

Risks

The risks of blood tests are minimal. These tests are not very accurate, however, and may cause unnecessary concern.

Diagnosis

Blood tests cannot confirm a specific diagnosis, but simply indicate the possibility of certain conditions, including neural tube defects such as spina bifida, and chromosomal problems such as Down syndrome. The woman may be offered a diagnostic test such as amniocentesis if her risk is high.

Stacey Chillemi's Experience

My doctors watched me closely while I was pregnant. I had blood tests to determine if I was on the right dosage of my AEDs, and ultrasounds to make sure the baby was developing normally. I also had level-2 ultrasounds, because they are more accurate. I have always preferred going to an epileptologist rather than a neurologist. After years of trying to find the right doctor, I realized that neurologists who do not specialize in epilepsy are not up-to-date on the new medicines, research, and ways of controlling seizures, because it is not their specialty. Epileptologists have a better understanding of how their patients feel and are able to relate to their patients better because they devote all of their time to their patients with epilepsy.

A survey of 3,535 health care professionals involved in the treatment of female patients with epilepsy revealed that information and awareness of health issues for female patients with epilepsy are usually low. The specialists included in the survey were family practitioners, obstetricians, epileptologists, and specialists in women's health and reproductive health. Only 5% of the survey respondents answered two thirds of the questions correctly. This lack of understanding points out the necessity of being your own advocate. Ask questions when you see your doctors and make sure you receive the best possible medical care.

Conclusions

GUIDELINES FOR PHYSICIANS AND OTHER HEALTH CARE PROFESSIONALS

1. Use the most effective antiepileptic drug in monotherapy at the lowest possible dose.

2. If there is a family history of neural tube defects and there are acceptable treatment alternatives, avoid valproate (Depakote) and carbamazepine (Tegretol).

3. Monitor the free (nonprotein-bound) fraction of the antiepileptic drug at each trimester, before delivery, and 4 to 8 weeks after delivery.

4. Adjust the antiepileptic drug dosage according to the nonprotein-bound (free) level.

5. Provide folate supplementation at a dosage of 0.4–4 mg per day before conception and throughout gestation.

6. Offer prenatal testing with anatomic ultrasound and maternal serum alpha-fetoprotein at 15 to 20 weeks of gestation.

7. Provide the pregnant woman with 10 mg of vitamin K per day during the last month of gestation, because antiepileptic medications can sometimes affect the level of vitamin K in the body. Vitamin K is necessary for normal clotting, and its lack in the mother can lead to risk of bleeding in the neonate.

GUIDELINES FOR PREGNANT WOMEN WITH EPILEPSY

Fortunately, there are many things you can do to ensure you have a healthy pregnancy and a healthy baby:

1. Take the vitamin supplements recommended by your doctors.

2. Tell the doctor about your family's medical history, and the history of family of the baby's father, including any brain or spinal defects.

3. Eat a healthy diet before, during, and after the pregnancy.

4. Limit or eliminate your caffeine intake.

5. Get sufficient sleep. It is normal to be tired during pregnancy, but when you are run-down you are more likely to have a seizure, so plenty of rest is important during pregnancy.

6. Exercise regularly. Exercising regularly helps keep you in shape, strengthens your body, and also relieves stress. Pregnancy is a joyous time, but it is a stressful time, too. Stress can cause seizures, so do whatever is necessary to make your pregnancy as stress-free as possible.

7. Avoid smoking, alcohol, and recreational drugs.

8. Take your AEDs as prescribed by your doctor.

9. Follow your doctor's recommendations regarding tests to rule out potential problems with the baby, including ultrasound and amniocentesis.

Early planning, management, and education are essential for all women of childbearing age who have epilepsy. Ultimately, a woman with epilepsy has the right to make an educated decision regarding pregnancy. The risk of having a baby with epilepsy or other problems often discourages couples from having children. If you are a woman with epilepsy and decide to conceive a child, you can use the strategies discussed in this book to increase your chances of having a normal pregnancy, birth, and baby.

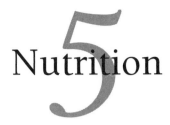

Nutrition

Even before pregnancy begins, nutrition is one of the most important factors in the health of a mother and her baby. If you are eating a well-balanced diet before you become pregnant, you will need to make only a few changes to meet the nutritional needs of pregnancy. Good quality nutrients form the foundation for healthy development of the baby. Pregnant women *must* eat well and should eat a wide range of foods in order to get the proper nutrients.

Doctors usually recommend general guidelines for a healthy diet during pregnancy, which include the basic nutrients necessary to meet the needs of the developing fetus. Avoid eating too much junk food, because it provides empty calories and insufficient nutrients.

Pregnancy is a good time to start eating right. A healthy diet is important for the following reasons:

❖ The baby will have a healthy birth weight.

❖ There is less risk that the baby will be born with infections or other problems.

❖ It reduces the risk for premature birth.

❖ It builds up fats and fluids in the mother's body for use during breast-feeding.

❖ It reduces the risk of complications during pregnancy.

Weight Gain

Weight gain during pregnancy should be gradual, with the most weight being gained in the last trimester. About 2 to 4 pounds should be gained during the first 3 months of pregnancy, and then 3 to 4 pounds per month for the rest of the pregnancy. Total weight gain should be about 25 to 30 pounds. This will decrease the risk of delivering a low-birth-weight baby.

Body Mass Index is an estimate of body composition based on height and weight; it is the ratio of the weight to the height squared. The Institute of Medicine recommends that women who have a low Body Mass Index should gain 28 to 40 pounds during pregnancy. Women who have a higher Body Mass Index should gain 15 to 25 pounds.

These weight gain estimates include 6 to 8 pounds for the weight of the baby. The remaining weight consists of higher fluid volume, larger breasts, larger uterus, amniotic fluid, and the placenta. Ask your doctor for an assessment of your weight gain throughout your pregnancy. The doctor can make recommendations about how much weight you should gain in order to ensure that your pregnancy is progressing smoothly, and make sure that you are getting the right amount of nutrients.

Fat deposits may increase by more than a third of the total amount a woman had before she became pregnant. If weight gain was normal during pregnancy, most women lose this extra weight during the birth process and in the weeks and months after birth. Breast-feeding helps to reduce the fat deposited during pregnancy. Women who breast-feed burn at least 500 more calories daily than women who do not, and should not be on a diet to lose weight. Poor maternal diet during breast-feeding can cause developmental, physical, and psychological problems in the child.

Women who do not gain enough weight have an increased risk for delivering babies with low birth weights (less than 5.52 pounds). The National Institutes of Health considers low birth weight a major public health problem in the United States. Low birth weight is a major cause of infant death, and babies who are underweight are at risk for physical and psychological childhood disorders. They are more likely to experience asthma, respiratory tract infections, and ear infections. Underweight babies—especially those who are born weighing less than 2.2 pounds—are at greater risk for cerebral palsy. They are more likely to score low on intelligence tests and be developmentally delayed.

Although infant death in the United States has declined over the past several decades, it is still a major public health problem. Among African Americans, about 13% of newborns are underweight; among Latinos, 6% to 9%; among Asian Americans, 5% to 8%; and among whites, approximately 6% of newborns are underweight. Racial variations in birth weight may reflect issues relating to economic development, poverty, health care reform, and general quality of life.

Varicose Veins

Gaining too much weight can make pregnancy an uncomfortable experience, causing backache, leg pain, and varicose veins. Varicose veins can occur anywhere there is increased pressure in a vein close to the skin, but they are most common in the legs and ankles. Varicose veins do not usually cause any symptoms, but when there are symptoms, they are often worse after prolonged sitting or standing, or late in the day.

Symptoms of varicose veins may include

❖ a dull, heavy aching or burning sensation and fatigue in the legs;

❖ mild swelling, usually in the feet and ankles;

❖ itchy skin over the varicose vein;

❖ bulging, twisted veins and a slight bluish outline of the vein that can be seen through the skin;

❖ sensitivity to touch;

❖ cramping in the legs, especially at nighttime; and

❖ bleeding in the skin over or in the region of the varicose vein.

Varicose veins are common, and they are usually not a serious medical problem. Women are usually most concerned about the way they look. Varicose veins can be treated at home using exercise, the wearing of elastic stockings, and elevating the legs periodically throughout the day. This is all most women with varicose veins need in order to find relief. Some women may choose to have a procedure that closes the vein, including sclerotherapy (injection of a chemical irritant), laser therapy, or surgery.

Dietary Guidelines

Pregnant women should increase their servings of the foods from the four basic food groups, including the following:

❖ Four or more servings of fruits and vegetables (for vitamins and minerals)

❖ Four or more servings of whole-grain or enriched bread and cereal (for energy)

❖ Four or more servings of milk and milk products (or calcium)

❖ Three or more servings of meat, poultry, fish, eggs, nuts, and dried beans and peas (for protein)

Most physicians agree that recommended daily allowances (RDA) can be obtained through a proper diet (except the RDA for iron). Table 5-1 outlines the recommended daily allowance for each age group, including those for pregnant women.

The nutritional requirements for pregnant women differ, depending on individual needs. Iron is needed in larger doses for the production of healthy red blood cells, especially during the later stages of pregnancy. It is difficult for a woman to consume enough iron from foods to maintain a sufficient supply, which often leaves her anemic and tired, and an iron supplement may be prescribed by the doctor. Anemia is a condition that develops when the blood is lacking in healthy red blood cells, the main transporter of oxygen to the organs. Anemia causes fatigue because of lack of oxygen.

TABLE 5-1
RECOMMENDED DAILY ALLOWANCES FOR ADULT FEMALES (by age)

Ages:	15–18	19–24	25–50	51+	Pregnant
Calories	2,200	2,200	2,200	1,900	+300
Protein	44	46	50	50	60
Vitamin E	8	8	8	8	10
Vitamin K	55	60	65	65	65
Vitamin C	60	60	60	60	70
Thiamin	1.1	1.1	1.1	1.0	1.5
Riboflavin	1.3	1.3	1.3	1.2	1.6
Niacin	15	15	15	13	17
Vitamin B_6	1.5	1.6	1.6	1.6	2.2
Folate	180	180	180	180	400
Vitamin B_{12}	2.0	2.0	2.0	2.0	2.2
Iron	15	15	15	10	30
Zinc	12	12	12	12	15
Selenium	50	55	55	55	65

Women of childbearing age are particularly susceptible to iron-deficiency anemia, because of the blood loss from menstruation and increased blood supply demands during pregnancy. Anemia can make women less able to fight off infections and unable to handle hemorrhaging during labor and delivery. Severe folic acid deficiency can result in megaloblastic anemia, which occurs most often in the last trimester of pregnancy. In this type of anemia—where the young, developing red cells in the bone marrow are large and abnormal—the mother's heart, liver, and spleen may become enlarged, threatening the life of the fetus. Folic acid can be found in many foods, including kidney beans, leafy green vegetables, peas, and liver. Women should consume plenty of these foods during their childbearing years. Folic acid is so important to the health of women and their babies that the Food and Drug Administration recently required the addition of folic acid to prepackaged breads and cereals.

What you eat and drink affects your baby. As stated previously, avoid drinking any alcoholic beverages while you are pregnant. Alcohol can cause fetal alcohol syndrome (FAS), a condition that can affect your baby for its entire life. FAS is a preventable cause of birth defects and mental retardation.

Caffeine is a stimulant found in colas, coffee, tea, chocolate, and many nonprescription and prescription medications. It can cause irritability, nervousness, and insomnia, as well as low-birth-weight babies when consumed in quantity. Caffeine is also a diuretic and can deprive the pregnant woman's body of valuable water. Some studies indicate that caffeine intake during pregnancy can harm the fetus, and it should be avoided as much as possible.

Other additions to the diet during pregnancy include the following:

❖ Calcium. Pregnant and lactating adult women require a 40% increase in calcium per day (1,200–1,500 mg per day). Almost all of the extra calcium goes into the baby's developing bones. To get enough calcium, three extra servings (3 cups) of milk or dairy products are needed. You can get extra calcium from low-lactose or reduced-lactose products if you are lactose intolerant, or your doctor may prescribe a calcium supplement.

❖ Sodium. Salt is important during pregnancy, and 2,000–8,000 mgs a day is recommended. There are 2,325 mgs of sodium in one teaspoon of salt and because salt is found in most foods, the increased need for it during pregnancy is easy to satisfy. Sodium helps to regulate the water in the body.

❖ Fluids. Drink plenty of fluids, especially water. A woman's blood volume increases dramatically during pregnancy. Drinking at least eight glasses of water a day can help prevent common problems such as dehydration and constipation.

The food cravings of pregnant women may reflect changes in their nutritional needs. These changes help guarantee normal development of the baby and satisfy the demands of breast-feeding after the baby is born.

The need for additional nutrients does not mean you need to eat twice as much! An increase of only 300 calories per day is recommended. For example, a baked potato has 120 calories, so getting those extra 300 calories should not be that difficult. Low-calorie intake can cause the mother's stored fat to break down, leading to the production of substances called ketones. The presence of ketones in the mother's blood and urine is a sign of starvation or a starvation-like state. Constant production of ketones can result in a child with mentally retardation.

Diabetes

Diabetic women should be closely monitored to make sure their blood sugar levels are normal or near normal. If the maternal blood sugar rises too high, the increased sugar crossing into the placenta can result in a large, overdeveloped baby with defects or blood sugar level abnormalities. Having a large baby can also result in injuries during birth and increase the need for cesarean delivery or other assistance during delivery, such as forceps or vacuum delivery. Women who are diabetic may also suffer from a greater loss of some nutrients. It is important to maintain tight control of blood sugar before and during pregnancy.

Gestational diabetes is a form of diabetes that begins during pregnancy. It usually disappears after the birth of the baby. Gestational diabetes is indicated by a high amount of sugar in the pregnant woman's blood. It is a relatively common problem, affecting 2% to 4% percent of all pregnant women. You are more likely to develop gestational diabetes if you

❖ are overweight when you become pregnant

❖ have high blood pressure or other medical complications

❖ have given birth to a large baby previously

❖ have given birth to a baby that was stillborn or had certain birth defects

❖ have had gestational diabetes previously

❖ have a family history of diabetes

❖ come from an African, Hispanic, Asian, Native American, or Pacific Islander ethnic background

❖ are more than 30 years old

Half of all women who develop gestational diabetes have no known risk factors. Gestational diabetes can cause severe complications for newborns if left untreated. The baby may have a greater chance of developing jaundice, a condition in which the skin and whites of the eyes turn yellowish in color. About half of all newborns develop mild jaundice in the first few days. In premature babies, jaundice may start early and last longer than in full-term babies.

The risk of birth defects in newborn babies whose mothers have gestational diabetes is very low, because in most cases this type of diabetes develops after the 20th week of pregnancy, when the fetus is already fully developed. The risk increases only if you had undiagnosed diabetes before pregnancy, or if you have high, uncontrolled blood sugar levels during the first 6 to 8 weeks of pregnancy.

Gestational diabetes in the mother is *not* a risk factor for the baby's developing type 1 diabetes during childhood. Type 1 diabetes is a lifelong disease that develops when the pancreas stops producing insulin. Insulin is a hormone that allows glucose (sugar) to move from the blood into the cells of the body, to be used for energy, or to be stored in the muscle, fat, and liver cells for later use. If glucose cannot move from the blood into the cells, the blood sugar will rise above a safe level and the cells will not be able to function properly.

Type 2 diabetes develops when the pancreas cannot produce enough insulin, or when the tissues of the body become resistant to insulin. Children borne to women who have gestational diabetes are more likely to develop type 2 diabetes later in life as well as be overweight throughout life.

Blood sugar levels rise so slowly in type 2 diabetes that a person usually does not have symptoms and may have had the disease for many years before diagnosis. If diabetes is not treated and blood sugar levels remain high for extended periods of time, the blood vessels and nerves throughout the body may be damaged, resulting in an increased risk for eye, heart, blood vessel, nerve, and kidney disease.

The common symptoms of diabetes include increased thirst, frequent urination, increased hunger, unusual weight loss, extreme fatigue, and irritability.

The blood sugar levels of most women return to normal after delivery. Once you have had gestational diabetes, however, you are more likely to develop it if you get pregnant again. You also have an increased risk of developing diabetes later in your life—there is a 50% chance of developing diabetes within 10 years of delivery. Type 2 diabetes can be controlled through diet management, medication, and exercise.

Morning Sickness

Morning sickness, nausea, occasional vomiting, tiredness, and exhaustion are common to about 70% of pregnant women. It is vital to manage morning sickness during your pregnancy, because vomiting can interfere with anti-epileptic drug intake, absorption, and compliance. Most nausea occurs during the first trimester and goes away during the second trimester. Morning sickness does not always happen in the morning. You can get morning sickness for no apparent reason, and at any time of day. For some women, it might last longer than the early stage of pregnancy. Some women experience morning sickness throughout the entire 9 months. No one understands exactly what causes morning sickness, but many factors are known to contribute to morning sickness, including low blood sugar, low blood pressure, hormonal changes, nutritional deficiencies (vitamin B6 and iron), nutritional excess (spicy, sugary, and refined foods), fatigue, and stress.

A study at Cornell University in New York suggested that morning sickness might have a helpful function. When researchers analyzed different studies involving more than 80,000 pregnancies, they found that nausea and vomiting are most common when the baby is going through its most sensitive period of development (the first trimester). Aversions to certain foods are common at this time—usually meat, fish, eggs, poultry, and strong-tasting vegetables.

According to researchers, nausea and vomiting may be the way the body gets rid of chemicals, bacteria, and food-borne and other types of illnesses that can be harmful to the mother and fetus. Researchers have also found that morning sickness is uncommon in cultures in which the diet is mainly vegetarian and in which dairy foods are not staples.

Many women worry that morning sickness is a sign that there is something wrong with the baby. This is not true. A study published in the *Journal of Obstetrics and Gynecology* observed that morning sickness is associated with better pregnancy outcomes, including a decreased risk of miscarriage, preterm birth, low birth weight, and perinatal death. Researchers also believe that morning sickness may support the healthy growth of the placenta, although they do not yet know how. This may be reassuring, though it does not help when you are feeling miserable.

Over the years, doctors have tried many medical solutions to morning sickness. One of the most disturbing was thalidomide, which is used to treat and prevent the debilitating and disfiguring skin sores associated with erythema nodosum leprosum (ENL), an inflammatory complication of leprosy. In the late 1950s and 1960s, however, pregnant women who took thalidomide gave birth to babies with severe deformities.

Since that time, doctors and midwives have been reluctant to prescribe any medications for the transient nausea so common in early pregnancy. They are not often effective, in any case. Most women are also reluctant to take medications for morning sickness. They prefer to look for natural methods.

Severe nausea accompanied by vomiting during pregnancy is rare, but requires medical attention because the body can become dehydrated and robbed of essential nutrients. Consult your doctor if nausea or vomiting is keeping you from eating right or gaining enough weight.

For the common nausea that is experienced by many pregnant women, try the following self-help remedies:

❖ Take 2 to 3 teaspoons of apple cider vinegar in warm water first thing in the morning. Apple cider vinegar is pH neutral, and may help to neutralize excess stomach acid.

❖ Ginger has been thoroughly researched, and may be taken freely. A review of the scientific evidence, published in the *British Journal of Anaesthesia*, found that ginger is beneficial in treating all kinds of nausea. Pour boiling water over a teaspoon of freshly grated ginger root to make a tea. You can also add the juice of half a lemon and sweeten with honey. Ginger tea is warming in the winter, and it can be a refreshing iced tea in the summer. This tea also wards off low blood sugar, headaches, and fatigue. If you are out of the house and cannot brew ginger tea, any food item containing ginger should help. Some women swear by stale ginger ale; others prefer the crystallized ginger that is available in some specialty shops. Ginger can also be used liberally in cooking both sweet and savory dishes.

❖ Acupressure can also be very effective. Several studies, including those published in the *Journal of the Royal Society of Medicine* and the *Journal of Nurse Midwifery*, show that pressure on the pericardium 6 (or P6) point can provide fairly quick relief from nausea, although it may not help to reduce vomiting. To find this point, place your hand palm up and measure two thumb widths above the most prominent wrist crease; P6 is just above this point, in line with your middle finger. Some drugstores sell wristbands that stimulate the P6 point; they have been shown to work for some women.

Nausea in early pregnancy is a condition that often can be remedied by taking care of your body nutritionally:

❖ Eat small meals.

❖ Do not skip meals or avoid going long periods without food.

❖ Drink fluids between meals, but not with meals.

❖ Avoid foods that are greasy, fried, or highly spiced.

❖ Avoid foul and unpleasant odors.

❖ Rest when you are tired.

Keeping Fit During Pregnancy

A lways check with your doctor before you begin any physical activity to make sure that it's safe for you to exercise during your pregnancy. Some questions have been raised about the effects of exercise on pregnant women, but there is no proof that gentle exercise has any negative effects. Studies have not shown any benefits for the baby, but exercise might help you feel better and maintain your weight. Exercise also helps prepare a woman for childbirth by strengthening the muscles and increasing vitality, and it will be much easier to get back into shape after the baby has been born. If you don't have any serious medical problems and you have an uncomplicated pregnancy, it is probably safe for you to do some exercising.

Your doctor may limit the amount or type of exercise you can do, or tell you not to exercise at all if you experience certain medical conditions, including the following:

❖ Preterm rupture of membranes

❖ Pregnancy-induced hypertension

❖ Preterm labor (A typical full-term pregnancy lasts 37 to 42 weeks, calculated from the first day of your last menstrual period to childbirth. Preterm labor, or premature labor, is the early onset of uterine contractions before 37 weeks, but after 20 weeks of pregnancy.)

❖ Persistent second or third trimester bleeding

❖ Poor fetal growth

❖ Incompetent cervix

❖ Multiple-birth pregnancy

If your doctor says it is okay, you can begin exercising at a degree that does not cause pain, shortness of breath, or excessive tiredness. You may then slowly increase your activity. If you feel uncomfortable, short of breath, or very tired, you should reduce your level of exercise. If you have already been exercising, it is easier to keep exercising during pregnancy. If you have not exercised before, you need to start very slowly. Many women find they need to decrease the amount of exercise they do during pregnancy.

Be careful to avoid activities that increase your risk of falls or injury, such as contact sports or vigorous sports. Even mild injuries to the "tummy" area can be serious when you're pregnant. After the first 3 months of pregnancy, it's best to avoid exercising while lying on your back, since the weight of the baby may interfere with blood circulation. Also, try to avoid long periods of standing.

When the weather is hot, exercise in the early morning or late evening so that you don't become worked up. If you are exercising indoors, make sure the room has enough ventilation. It is a good idea to keep yourself cool and perhaps to have a portable fan by your side. Drink plenty of fluids, even if you do not feel thirsty, and make sure that you are eating a well-balanced diet. Normally, pregnancy increases your food requirements by 300 calories a day, even without exercise.

Staying active during pregnancy does not necessarily mean you have to overexert yourself until your muscles start to ache. Your body releases a hormone called relaxin during pregnancy that loosens your joints in preparation for delivery, so avoid strenuous exercise.

Make sure you drink plenty of water prior to, during, and after exercising, especially when the weather is hot or humid. You do not have to feel dehydrated to actually be dehydrated. An increase in core body temperature during early pregnancy can cause fetal defects; dehydration in late pregnancy can cause premature labor.

Stacey Chillemi's Experience

I always had seizures if I spent too much time outside in the hot, humid weather. It was summer when I was pregnant with my son Michael, but even though I enjoy summer, I spent it inside the house, where there was air conditioning. I didn't want to take any chances, because I wasn't just worrying about just myself anymore; I had the baby to consider.

General Safety Guidelines for Exercising

1. Always start your exercise with a warm-up, and end with a cool-down. Gentle stretches will prevent strains, joint injuries, and muscle cramps.

2. Wear comfortable clothes when exercising. Your choice of clothing can also help you keep cool. Wear shoes that have good cushioning under the heel in order to avoid injuries to the foot or Achilles tendon, which connects the calf muscle to the heel bone. It is the largest tendon in the human body, and withstands a large amount of force with each foot movement. The Achilles tendon allows the foot to point downward and enables you to stand on your toes.

3. Wear a sports bra or a support bra with side adjustment straps for good support during exercise, because the breasts become sensitive during pregnancy.

4. If you experience any symptoms such as chest pains, vaginal bleeding, or uterine contractions, or if your membranes rupture, stop exercising immediately and call your doctor.

5. If possible, eat five or six small meals or snacks per day to replace the calories used during exercise.

6. Avoid exercising on your back after the first trimester, or whenever you feel dizzy, lightheaded, or nauseated. The weight of the uterus puts pressure on the vein responsible for returning blood from the lower body to the heart. Also, do not stand for long periods of time.

7. Avoid contact sports such as football and basketball; adventure sports such as water skiing and scuba diving; and sports that carry a high risk of trauma such as horseback riding and downhill skiing.

8. Do not overflex or overextend the knee joints (as in deep-knee bends) unless your body is well conditioned for these motions. Knee joints are more prone to injury during pregnancy because the ligaments and tendons are softened.

9. Exercise gets your heart pumping, keeps your body flexible, helps you control weight gain, and gets your muscles ready for the hard work of labor and delivery—without causing unnecessary stress

on your body or the baby. Many activities, such as running, are fine in early pregnancy, but you may need to adjust your exercise regimen as your body becomes larger. Avoid activities that could put you at risk for slips and falls, such as bicycling, rollerblading, horseback riding, and skiing. Even mild injuries to the abdomen can be serious when you are pregnant.

Exercises for Pregnancy

The following exercises are reasonably safe for pregnant women, even though some of them may not be advisable during the third trimester. Always consult your doctor for advice regarding your specific situation.

WALKING

Walking is one of the best cardiovascular exercises for pregnant women, because it tones the muscles, gets you to get out of the house and breathing fresh air, and promotes good sleep. It keeps you fit without hurting your knees and ankles, is safe for the entire 9 months of pregnancy, and is an easy way to begin exercising if you have been sedentary.

Continue your regular walking program, or begin by walking for 20 to 30 minutes per day 3 days a week. Slowly increase to 30 to 60 minutes on most, if not all, days of the week.

Tips for Walking During the First Trimester

Wear proper walking shoes so that your feet get the support they need, particularly around the ankles and arches. Wear a sun hat and carry a spray bottle of water for cooling off during the summer. The heat from the sun can drain you and stress your body to the point that you become prone to having a seizure. Bring drinking water with you to prevent dehydration. Consider mall walking as an alternative during hot weather. (But do not spend too much money while you are at the mall!)

Do not push yourself to the extreme. Your pulse rate should not be above 140 beats per minute at any time during your walk. You should be able to speak in complete sentences without gasping for breath. A pulse of more than 100 beats per minute 5 minutes after a workout means you have worked your body too hard.

Tips for Walking During the Second Trimester

You will start to become clumsy when walking during the second trimester because your body is expanding. Pay attention to your posture when you walk in order to avoid straining your back. Keep your head straight, chin level, hips tucked under your shoulders to avoid swayback, and your eyes on what lies ahead. Swing your arms for balance and to increase your workout. Walking with a friend will keep you motivated.

Tips for Walking During the Third Trimester

Keep up your walking routine as long as you can, but avoid vigorous activities, such as hiking on steep trails, mountain climbing, or walking on uneven land that could put you off-balance. As you get closer to your due date, you may also want to consider walking on a track. The surface will be easier on your body, and you will feel safe knowing that you are not far from home or your car in case of an emergency.

Safety Guidelines for Walking

Never walk to the point of exhaustion or breathlessness. Pushing yourself to the limit forces your body to use oxygen that should be going to your baby. Stop walking immediately and call your doctor as soon as possible if you have any of the following symptoms: vaginal bleeding, dizziness, fainting, blurred vision, contractions.

JOGGING/RUNNING

If you enjoy jogging or running, you probably will want to continue doing so during your pregnancy. Jogging and running are safe activities, and many pregnant women continue them, with modification, throughout pregnancy. If you have never run before, however, now is not a good time to start.

Running is the quickest way to work your heart and body, giving you a mental, physical, and spiritual boost. It is easy to fit jogging or running into your schedule—running 15 minutes one day when that is all you have time for, and a half hour when your schedule permits.

If you are the type of person who laces up your sneakers and runs out the door without stretching, it is time to change your ways! Now that you are pregnant, you need to take some extra safety measures. Stretching before and after running will help prevent injuries. Gentle, easy stretching is best.

Slow down to a walk if you feel Braxton Hicks contractions (rhythmic tightening of the lower abdomen) or ligament pain. Stop exercising and consult your doctor if you feel any type of pain, persistent contractions, leakage of fluid, fatigue, dizziness, or anything else unusual.

Tips for Jogging/Running During the First Trimester

During the first trimester, you may experience bouts of nausea and fatigue. Try running outdoors if you normally run on an indoor track. The fresh air may help. If you find yourself losing weight because of vomiting, cut back or stop exercising until you are gaining adequate weight.

The first few months of pregnancy can be difficult, because you will probably begin to feel fatigue. Run during the day when you feel the least tired. Running with tender swollen breasts is uncomfortable. As the weeks go by, you may need to move up to a larger size bra.

You will begin to urinate more frequently during the first trimester. Try to run close to home so that you will be near the bathroom. Make sure you stop any racing, speed work, or vigorous long runs once you learn you are pregnant.

Tips for Jogging/Running During the Second Trimester

Your center of gravity shifts during the second trimester as your belly grows, leaving you at risk for slips and falls. Jog or run on flat pavement for safety. Try to fall correctly if you do lose your balance: fall to your side or on your buttocks, to avoid trauma to the abdomen. You may want to start running on a track as your pregnancy progresses.

Tips for Jogging/Running During the Third Trimester

If you feel too fatigued to go for a run, listen to your body and take a break. Although being inactive is unhealthy, pushing yourself too hard is also harmful. Most avid runners find that their pace slows down considerably during the third trimester—a fast waddle or shuffle may be the most they can manage.

SWIMMING

Doctors and fitness experts agree that swimming is the most beneficial and safest exercise for pregnant women. Swimming exercises the large muscle groups of the arms and legs and provides good cardiovascular benefits, even though it is low impact. Swimming allows you to feel weightless despite the extra pounds of pregnancy. It is also a very safe form of exercise because the risk of injury is low. If you swam a lot before you got pregnant, you should be able to continue without too much change in your regimen. If you did not exercise at all, you should still be able to start swimming. You will need to start slowly, stretch well before and after, and warm up and cool down gradually.

Tips for Swimming During the First Trimester

If you have the energy, swim for at least 20 minutes every other day for the greatest benefit. Swimming first thing in the morning may relieve morning sickness and fatigue.

Tips for Swimming During the Second Trimester

You will not have to cut down on swimming as your body grows larger. You probably will not need to adjust your schedule, but wearing a maternity swimsuit may be more comfortable as your belly expands. It may be difficult to find one, however, if it is off-season. Try going to a maternity shop or shopping on the Internet.

Tips for Swimming During the Third Trimester

The water will support your joints and ligaments as you swim, preventing injury. You will not get overheated when swimming. The breaststroke is particularly beneficial in the third trimester, because it lengthens the chest muscles and shortens the back muscles, two areas that typically become uneven as your body changes during pregnancy. Use a snorkel to relieve the pressure on your neck that is created when turning your head to breathe.

AEROBIC EXERCISE

Aerobic exercise helps increase the ability of the body to process and use oxygen, which is important for you and your baby. Aerobic exercise also has the following benefits:

- ❖ Improves circulation
- ❖ Increases muscle tone and strength

❖ Builds stamina

❖ Burns calories

❖ Builds strength and is energizing

❖ Promotes good sleep

❖ Conditions the body to cope with the physical and emotional challenges of pregnancy

An aerobics class provides a consistent time slot when you know you will exercise. If you sign up for a class specifically designed for pregnant women, you will also enjoy the camaraderie of other women. Many community recreation centers offer prenatal exercise classes. If you already attend a regular aerobics class, let your instructor know that you are pregnant. The instructor will suggest ways to modify any movements that may be unsafe or too strenuous. An aerobic exercise video may be helpful if you prefer to exercise at home.

Aerobic exercise strengthens the heart and lungs, and helps maintain muscle tone. As long as you choose exercises that are low-impact—and keep one foot on the ground at all times to minimize stress on your joints—you should be able to continue exercising throughout your pregnancy.

YOGA AND STRETCHING

There are many benefits to be gained from the practice of yoga. It can help you mentally and physically during your pregnancy, and it is also beneficial for the physical and mental development of the fetus. Yoga helps ensure an optimum supply of blood and nutrients to the developing fetus, and can ensure a smooth pregnancy and a relatively easy childbirth. The authors recommend consulting a good basic yoga book for details on the positions that will be discussed and working with an experienced yoga instructor.

Yoga and stretching can help maintain muscle tone and flexibility with little or no impact on your joints. Yoga also improves balance and circulation. Prenatal yoga classes are very popular with pregnant women. Being in a positive, supportive environment can give you a regular emotional boost, and keep you motivated to continue exercising.

Yoga and stretching—when combined with a cardiovascular exercise such as walking—is an ideal way to maintain fitness while you are pregnant. Yoga and stretching are helpful for the following:

1. Relieving fluid retention and cramping, which are quite common during pregnancy

2. Influencing the position of the baby, and turning it in advance of labor, if needed

3. Stimulating bowel action and appetite

4. Raising energy levels while also slowing the metabolism

5. Relaxation

6. Reducing nausea, morning sickness, and mood swings when exercises are performed in combination with yogic breathing called *pranayama*

7. Relieving tension around the cervix and birth canal

8. Focusing on opening the pelvis to make labor easier and quicker

Yoga also helps women adjust to the physical demands of labor, birth, and motherhood. One of the first things you learn in a yoga class is how to breathe fully, using a breathing technique called *ujayi*. This technique requires you to take in air slowly through your nose, filling your lungs entirely, and then exhaling completely until your stomach compresses. Learning how to do ujayi breathing primes you for labor and childbirth by training you to stay calm when you need it the most. When you are afraid (during labor, for example), the body produces adrenalin and shuts down the production of oxytocin, a hormone that makes labor progress. Yogic training will help you fight the urge to tighten up when you experience labor pain, and will teach you how to relax using breathing.

Tips for Practicing Yoga During the First Trimester

Seek out instructors who are specially trained in prenatal yoga, but if that is not possible, make sure your instructor knows that you are expecting. Tell the instructor how far along you are in your pregnancy. There are few restrictions during the first trimester, but remember to follow these general safety guidelines:

❖ Drink plenty of water before, during, and after yoga practice.

❖ Breathe deeply and regularly.

❖ Modify your routine as your pregnancy progresses.

❖ Avoid overexertion.

❖ Stop immediately if you feel pain or discomfort.

Safety Guidelines for Doing Yoga During Pregnancy

Incorporate the following safety measures into any yoga program:

1. Be aware that your slowly expanding girth affects your sense of balance.

2. Avoid holding poses for lengthy periods of time.

3. Sink into the postures slowly and carefully in order to avoid injury.

4. Do not push your body beyond reasonable limits.

5. Avoid any movements that require you to be in a lying-down position. This position can result in vena cava syndrome, a condition in which blood flow to the uterus is decreased. Some women do not experience this syndrome and are comfortable lying down well into their pregnancies.

6. Avoid the head or shoulder stand if you have not done them before, although women who are familiar with these poses can continue to do them well into their second trimester. Avoid them completely during the third trimester.

7. Avoid positions that stretch the abdominal muscles too much, such as deep forward and back bends.

Stretches

The following eight stretches will enhance your flexibility, prevent your muscles from tightening, and make you look and feel great. Use them after a workout as a way to cool down, or when you need to relax. Be sure to breathe deeply and regularly as you stretch.

Shoulder circles (may be done standing or seated)

1. Rotate your shoulders forward, up, back, and down in the largest circle you can make.

2. Reverse the direction.

3. Repeat 4 times in each direction.

Arm stretch

1. Stand and interlace your fingers behind your lower back.

2. Pull your arms up as far as they can go toward the ceiling, and then lower them toward your buttocks.

3. Release and repeat 8–10 times.

Standing back stretch (You may want to avoid this stretch when you get too large to bend over comfortably.)

1. Stand with your feet about 12 inches apart.

2. Bend your knees slightly while rolling your head and torso forward and down, one vertebra at a time, toward the floor.

3. Return to a standing position by slowly rolling back up, one vertebra at a time, and straightening your knees. (Keep your weight centered on both feet.)

4. Repeat 8–10 times.

Waist twist

1. Stand with your feet shoulder-width apart for stability.

2. Extend both of your arms toward your left side while looking over your right shoulder.

3. Repeat the motion while looking over your left shoulder.

4. Increase your speed so your arms swing from side to side. Do not get carried away, however. You may lose your balance if you swing too quickly.

Wall push-up and calf stretch

1. Stand about 2 feet from a wall with your arms extended forward in front of your shoulders.

2. Reach your hands to the wall and lean forward, bending your elbows as your body tilts.

3. Keep your heels on the floor to stretch your calf muscles. (Do not do this exercise in socks or slippery shoes; your feet should remain stable.)

4. Push slowly away from the wall to straighten up.

5. Repeat 8–10 times.

Sitting back stretch

1. Sit on the floor with your legs stretched out parallel in front of you.

2. Slowly drop your head toward your knees and stretch your fingers along your legs as far as they will comfortably go. As your belly gets larger you will need to make adjustments.

3. Sit up slowly. Repeat 8–10 times.

Thigh stretch

1. Sit on the floor with your legs stretched out parallel in front of you.

2. Cross your right ankle over your left knee.

3. Use your left hand to pull your right thigh toward the left, stretching the outside of the right leg.

4. Increase the twist by looking over your right shoulder. Hold for one minute.

5. Repeat 8–10 times. Switch sides. You will have to make adjustments as your abdomen gets larger. Do what feels comfortable.

Leg stretch

1. Lie on your left side with your head on a pillow or folded towel.

2. Bend your left leg at the knee while keeping your right leg straight. Use your right hand as a brace on the floor in front of you.

3. Stretch your right leg as you lift it toward the ceiling, and then lower it to the floor.

4. Repeat 4 times, and then switch sides.

DANCE

You can get your heart pumping by dancing to your favorite tunes in the comfort and privacy of your living room, but avoid break-dancing or other dance movements that call for leaping, jumping, or twirling. You can lose yourself in music and stay fit. Think about signing up for a dance class.

Besides the thrill of moving through space, dancing is a great way to keep flexible while toning your muscles at the same time. You can get an aerobic workout from jazz or other fast-paced dance, or stretch and maintain muscle tone when you hold positions in ballet. Dance for at least 20 minutes three times a week for maximum benefit, whether it is in your living room or in a class.

Tips for Dancing During the First Trimester

Dance as you normally would, but keep a few precautions in mind. Warm up beforehand to prepare your joints and muscles for exercise and to help build up your heart rate slowly. As a general rule, your heart rate should not exceed 140 beats per minute (this number may vary depending on your level of fitness). Adjust the intensity of your dancing according to how you feel. Slow down if you are not able to carry on a conversation comfortably while dancing. Keep your workout impact low by leaving one foot on the floor at all times, substituting marching in place for jumps, or stepping side-to-side. Be aware of the limitations of your body.

Tips for Dancing During the Second and Third Trimesters

Avoid jumping, jarring motions, or quick changes in direction to prevent injuries to your ankles, knees, and ligaments. Jumps, lifts, dip, and fast spins are also off-limits.

KEGEL EXERCISES

The muscles in your pelvis will become stronger if you practice the Kegel exercise, also referred to as "pelvic floor exercise." Practicing Kegels on a regular basis will help develop the tone and flexibility of your pelvic floor muscles in preparation for delivery. It will also help the muscles return to normal after delivery.

The Kegel exercise involves tightening the two major muscles that stretch across the pelvic floor—the hammock and the triangle muscles. It is important to make sure that you use only these muscles. Be careful not to tighten your stomach, leg, or other muscles. Squeezing the wrong muscles can put more pressure on your bladder. Avoid holding your breath.

There are three methods to help locate the correct muscles:

1. Sit on the toilet and start to urinate. Try to stop the flow of the
    urine halfway through by contracting your pelvic floor muscles.
    Repeat this several times until you become familiar with con-
    tracting the right group of muscles.

2. Imagine that you are trying to stop passing gas. Squeeze the
    muscles that you would use. If you feel a pulling sensation, you
    have found the correct muscles for this exercise.

3. Lie down and put your finger inside your vagina. Squeeze as if
    you were trying to stop urinating. If you feel tightness on your
    finger, you are squeezing the correct pelvic muscles.

After you have identified the pelvic muscles, you can do the following
exercise on a regular basis as long as it is comfortable. Find a quiet, relaxing
place to practice this exercise:

1. Lie on the floor.

2. Squeeze your pelvic muscles and slowly count from 1 to 10. Then
    slowly release the muscles for 3 seconds.

3. Work up to 10–15 repetitions each time you exercise.

4. Practice these exercises several times a day until you are doing
    several sets of 10.

You can do Kegels while lying on the floor, sitting at a desk, or
standing in the kitchen. Practice this exercise at least three times a day
using all three positions in order to make your muscles even stronger.

Fetal Development

Pregnancy is a miraculous experience that will change you forever. It changes the way you observe life, and the way you relate to your family and friends. During the 9 months of pregnancy, you will grow spiritually and emotionally, as well as physically.

At the beginning of your menstrual cycle, approximately 20 ova (eggs) begin to develop in fluid-filled sacs called follicles. During the time you are fertile (approximately day 14 of your cycle), one (or more) of these follicles will mature and rupture, releasing an egg that will travel down the fallopian tube to the uterus, where it will await fertilization. After you conceive, your obstetrician will calculate when your pregnancy began by counting from the first day of your last menstrual period.

A sac begins to grow around the fertilized egg, which gradually fills with fluid and helps to cushion the growing embryo. This amniotic sac will break just prior to delivery, and the amniotic fluid will leak or gush out. When pregnant women say their water broke, they are referring to the bursting of the amniotic sac.

The placenta also begins to develop. This organ nourishes the fetus and produces the hormones that sustain pregnancy. It is attached to the wall of the uterus by arteries that supply it with maternal blood and oxygen.

The fetus is attached to the placenta by the umbilical cord, which is filled with blood vessels. These blood vessels transport blood, oxygen, and nutrients to the fetus, and carry away waste products and carbon dioxide. The mother's blood circulates on one side of the placenta; the fetal blood circulates on the other side. The mother's blood and the fetal blood do not mix.

The following is a description of fetal development by week:

Three weeks: The embryo is very small—about the size of the head of a pin. It does not resemble a fetus or baby; it is simply a group of approximately 100 cells that are multiplying and growing quickly. The outer layer of cells will become the placenta; the inner layer will become the embryo.

Four weeks: The embryo is still very small—about 0.014–0.04 inches. The embryo, probably in about its second week of development, has multiplied to approximately 150 cells. Secretions from the uterine lining nourish the embryo. The layers of cells are already specialized according to function. The outer layer will become the nervous system, skin, and hair; the inner layer will become the lungs and digestive organs; and the middle layer will become the skeleton, bones, cartilage, muscles, circulatory system, kidneys, and sex organs. The embryo's facial features continue to develop. Each ear begins as a little fold of skin at the side of the head. The tiny buds that will eventually grow into arms and legs are forming, as are fingers, toes, and eyes. The neural tube (brain, spinal cord, and other neural tissues of the central nervous system) is well formed. The digestive tract and sensory organs are beginning to develop. Bone starts to replace cartilage.

Five weeks: The embryo is approximately 0.05 inches. The heart, brain, spinal cord, muscle, and bones are beginning to develop. The placenta and the amniotic sac are still forming.

Six weeks: The embryo has begun to resemble a tadpole. It measures approximately 0.08–0.16 inches from the top of the head to the buttocks, and is about the size of a small pea. (This crown-to-rump length is used more often than crown-to-heel length because a fetus's legs are usually bent and therefore are hard to measure.) The eyes and limb buds are forming, and the heartbeat can sometimes be detected by ultrasound. This is an extremely important time in fetal development, because between 17 to 56 days the embryo is the most susceptible to factors that can interfere with normal growth.

Seven weeks: The embryo is now approximately 0.16–0.2 inches from crown to rump. It has a tiny beating heart. The embryo makes great strides in size this week, growing to 0.44–0.52 inches from crown to rump—about the size of a small raspberry. The leg buds are starting to resemble short fins, and the hands and feet have a digital plate where the fingers and toes will develop. The heart and lungs are becoming more developed, as are the eyes, nostrils, intestines, and appendix. The brain and spinal cord are growing from the neural tube.

Eight weeks: The embryo is approximately 0.56–0.8 inches from crown to rump—the size of a grape tomato. Eyelid folds and ears are forming, and the tip of the nose may be visible on ultrasound. The arms have grown longer and bend at the elbows. The places where the embryo's fingers and toes eventually will grow are becoming uneven. By the end of 8 weeks, the embryo will have distinct, slightly webbed fingers. The embryo's veins can now be seen, and the heart has divided into right and left chambers.

Nine weeks: The embryo measures approximately 0.9 inch–1.2 inches from crown to rump and is about the size of a lime. The arms and legs are longer, and the fingers might be a little swollen where the touch pads are forming. The head is becoming straight and the neck is more developed, but you will not be able to feel the embryo moving yet.

Ten weeks: The developing embryo is now officially called a fetus. It measures approximately 1.25–1.68 inches from crown to rump and weighs a little less than 0.2 ounces. The eyes are covered by skin that will eventually split to form eyelids.

Eleven weeks: The fetus measures approximately 1.75–2.4 inches from crown to rump and weighs about 0.3 ounces. It is about the size of a large lime. The rapid heartbeat can be heard through a Doppler sound-wave stethoscope. The fetus's fingernails and external genitalia now show distinguishing characteristics, and the fetus swallows and kicks. Unfortunately, at this point you still will not feel the fetus kicking or making other movements.

Twelve weeks: The fetus measures 2.5–3 inches from crown to rump and weighs 0.3–0.7 ounces. The fetus is entirely formed, and it will continue to get larger and stronger for the rest of the pregnancy. The chance of miscarriage drops significantly after 3 months, because the most important part of the fetus's development is complete at this point.

The fetus now has arms, hands, fingers, feet, and toes, and can open and close its fists and mouth. The external ears are formed, and the teeth are beginning to form. The circulatory and urinary systems are functioning, and the liver is producing bile. The eyelids, eyebrows, eyelashes, nails, and hair are formed. The teeth and bones have become denser. The fetus can even suck its thumb, yawn, stretch, and make faces. The nervous system is beginning to function. The reproductive organs and genitalia are now fully developed, and ultrasound can show whether it is a boy or a girl.

Thirteen weeks: The fully formed fetus measures 2.6–3.1 inches from crown to rump and weighs 0.5–0.7 ounces. It is about the size of a peach. The head is still larger than the body, but the rest of the body is starting to catch up. The fetus is growing very quickly at this point. The face is starting to look more human, with the eyes moving closer together. The toes and fingers are clearly separate, and the ankles and wrists have formed. The intestines are shifting into their proper place.

Fourteen weeks: The fetus measures about 3.2–4.1 inches from crown to rump and weighs almost 1 ounce. The ears are shifting from the neck to the sides of the head, and the neck is becoming longer and the chin more prominent. The fetus has facial features and unique fingerprints. The fetus is beginning to respond to outside movements and sounds such as voices, and will try to wiggle away if the mother's abdomen is poked.

Fifteen weeks: The fetus measures approximately 4.1–4.5 inches from crown to rump and weighs about 1.75 ounces. The eyebrows and the hair on the top of the head are beginning to grow. The bones are getting harder.

Sixteen weeks: The fetus measures approximately 4.3–4.6 inches from crown to rump and weighs about 2.8 ounces. The arms and legs are moving. The nervous system is functioning, and the muscles respond to stimulation from the brain. The skin is covered with a whitish coating called *vernix caseosa*. This "cheesy" substance—thought to protect the skin from exposure to the amniotic fluid—is shed just before birth. You may begin to feel the fetus move at this time. The first movement is called quickening. By the end of 4 months, the fetus is covered with a layer of thick, downy hair called lanugo, which is usually shed by the end of the first week after birth. The heartbeat can be heard clearly.

Seventeen weeks: The fetus measures approximately 4.4–4.8 inches from crown to rump and is now about 3.5 ounces. Fat is beginning to form, helping with heat production and metabolism. The lungs are beginning to exhale amniotic fluid, and the circulatory and urinary systems are working. Hair on the head, eyebrows, and eyelashes is thickening.

Eighteen weeks: The fetus measures approximately 5–5.6 inches from crown to rump and weighs approximately 5.25 ounces. Growth is beginning to slow down, but the reflexes are getting stronger. The developing fetus can now yawn, stretch, and make facial expressions, even frown. Taste buds are beginning to develop, and the fetus can tell the difference between sweet and bitter, and suck if its lips are stroked. It can swallow and even get the hiccups. The retinas have become sensitive to light, so if a bright light is shined on the abdomen the fetus may move to protect its eyes.

Nineteen weeks: The fetus measures approximately 5.2–6 inches from crown to rump and weighs about 7 ounces. The skin appears red because it is transparent and the blood vessels can be seen through it.

Twenty weeks: The fetus measures approximately 5.6–6.4 inches from crown to rump and weighs about 9 ounces. It may respond to sounds such as the mother's voice, heart, and her growling stomach, as well as sounds outside her body. It will cover its ears with its hands if a loud sound is made close by, and it may even become scared and do a little hop, skip, and jump. The fetus has become quite active by this time, moving often: twisting, turning, wiggling, punching, and kicking.

Twenty-one weeks: The fetus measures approximately 7.2 inches from crown to rump and weighs about 10.5 ounces. The fetus is steadily gaining fat. The growth rate is slowing down, but the various organ systems are continuing to mature. Buds for permanent teeth are beginning to form.

Twenty-two weeks: The fetus now measures approximately 7.6 inches and weighs about 12.3 ounces. The muscles are getting stronger, and the eyelids and eyebrows are developed. Movements are quite stable, and because the fetus now responds to sound, rhythm, and melody, you can try singing and talking to it. These same sounds will have a calming effect on the baby after it is born.

Twenty-three weeks: The fetus is now approximately 8 inches from crown to rump and weighs almost 1 pound. The body is becoming proportioned and is beginning to resemble a newborn, but the skin is still wrinkled because more weight needs to be gained. The lanugo may have turned darker.

Twenty-four weeks: The developing fetus measures approximately 8.4 inches from crown to rump and weighs about 1.2 pounds. It is starting to produce white blood cells for fighting disease and infection. It may respond to your touch or to sounds, and you may feel hiccups.

By the end of 24 weeks, the fetus has fingers and toe prints. The eyebrows and eyelids may be seen on ultrasound. The lungs are filled with amniotic fluid, and it has started making breathing motions. The eyelids begin to part and the eyes open. The fetus may respond to sounds by moving or increasing its pulse rate, and you may notice jerking motions from hiccups. The fetus may survive after 23 weeks of gestation with intensive care if born prematurely.

Twenty-five weeks: The fetus measures approximately 8.8 inches from crown to rump and weighs 1.5 pounds. The skin is thicker and no longer transparent. The heartbeat can be heard through a stethoscope, or depending on the position of the fetus, by others by putting their ear against your belly.

Twenty-six weeks: The fetus measures approximately 9.2 inches from crown to rump and weighs almost 2 pounds. Its hearing is fully developed. As it reacts to sounds, its pulse rate increases. The fetus will even move in rhythm to music. The lungs are still growing, but they are not yet mature. Patterns in the fetus's brain waves appear similar to those of a full-term newborn. The fetus also has its own individual patterns of sleeping and waking.

Twenty-seven weeks: The fetus measures approximately 9.6 inches from crown to rump and weighs a little more than 2 pounds. The hands are active, and muscle coordination is such that the fetus can get its thumb into its mouth. Thumb sucking calms the fetus and strengthens the cheek and jaw muscles. The fetus can cry by 27 weeks.

Twenty-eight weeks: The fetus measures approximately 10 inches from crown to rump, or a total length of about 15.75 inches from head to toe, and weighs about 2.4 pounds. Brain waves show rapid eye movement (REM) sleep, which means the fetus may be dreaming. The eyelids are opening. Branches of the fetus's lungs are developing, so there is a good chance that the fetus would survive if born prematurely at 28 weeks. By the end of 28 weeks, the body is well formed and fingernails cover the fingertips.

During the last 3 months of your pregnancy, your epileptologist will put you on vitamin K. Vitamin K is important for the prevention of blood clotting. Antiepileptic drugs can sometimes affect the level of vitamin K in your body. It is usually suggested to take 10 mg of Vitamin K1 daily during the last month of your pregnancy. This helps to decrease the danger of bleeding problems in the fetus during and after labor. It is important and so is suggested that the baby be given in injection of 1 mg of vitamin K1 when it is born.

Twenty-nine weeks: The fetus measures approximately 10.4 inches from crown to rump, or a total length of approximately 16.7 inches from head to toe, and weighs about 2.7 pounds. At this stage, the eyes of the fetus are almost always blue, and the fetus can distinguish bright sunlight or artificial light through the uterine wall. The fetus still does a lot of kicking and stretching.

Thirty weeks: The fetus measures approximately 17 inches from head to toe and weighs about 3 pounds. The fetus is getting fatter, and beginning to control its own body temperature. The eyebrows and eyelashes are fully developed, and the hair on the fetus's head is getting thicker.

Thirty-one weeks: The fetus measures approximately 18 inches from head to toe and weighs about 3.5 pounds. Rather than hearing vibrations, the nerve endings in the fetus's ears are connected now and it can hear distinct sounds such as familiar voices and music. The brain is developing rapidly at this time, and most of the internal systems are well developed, but the lungs may still be immature. The fetus may begin to move into a head-down position in preparation for birth.

Thirty-two weeks: The fetus measures approximately 18.9 inches from head to toe and weighs almost 4 pounds. The fetus will fill almost all of the space in the uterus by now, either lying with the head up or sometimes still with enough room to move around. A layer of fat is forming underneath the fetus's thin, wrinkly skin.

Thirty-three weeks: The fetus measures approximately 19.4 inches from head to toe and weighs about 4.4 pounds. The fetus will gain more than half its birth weight in the next 7 weeks. The fetus begins to move less now because it is running out of room. Instead, it will curl up with its knees bent, chin resting on its chest, and arms and legs crossed.

Thirty-four weeks: The fetus measures approximately 19.8 inches from head to toe and weighs about 5 pounds. The fetus is probably settling into the head-down position, although this change might not be complete. The organs are now almost fully mature, except for the lungs, and the skin is pink instead of red. Fingernails reach the ends of the fingers, but the toenails are not yet fully grown. The fetus might have abundant hair.

Thirty-five weeks: The fetus measures approximately 20.25 inches from head to toe, and weighs more than 5.5 pounds. The lungs are almost fully developed, but the fetus would probably need an incubator if it were born now, because it still does not have enough fat to keep warm outside of the womb. The fetus's reflexes are coordinated by this time, and it can blink, close its eyes, turn its head, grasp firmly, and respond to sounds, light, and touch. You should still feel movement every day by 35 weeks. The fetus's change in position continues in preparation for labor and delivery. The fetus drops down in the pelvis, with the head facing down toward the birth canal.

Thirty-six weeks: The fetus measures approximately 20.7 inches from head to toe and weighs about 6 pounds. The brain has been developing rapidly, and the fetus is practicing blinking.

Thirty-seven weeks: The fetus measures approximately 21 inches from head to toe and weighs almost 6.5 pounds. The fetus is getting rounder every day, and its skin is getting pinker and losing its wrinkly appearance. The head is usually positioned down into the pelvis by this time.

Thirty-eight weeks: The fetus measures approximately 21 inches from head to toe, and weighs about 6.8 pounds. Most of the fetus's lanugo and vernix are disappearing. The fetus is receiving antibodies from the mother to protect against illness. The fetus's growth is slowing, but the fat cells under the skin are getting thicker in preparation for life outside the womb. The fetus would do well if born at this time.

Thirty-nine weeks: The fetus measures approximately 21.5 inches from head to toe and weighs a little more than 7 pounds. The toenails have grown to the tips of the toes. The muscles of the fetus's arms and legs are strong, and it practices lung movements.

Forty weeks: The fetus measures approximately 21.5 inches from head to toe and weighs about 7.5 pounds. Boys often tend to weigh a little more than girls do. More lanugo falls out, but some may remain at birth on the shoulders, the folds of skin, and the backs of the ears.

By the end of your pregnancy, the fetus is about 8 pounds and measures between 18 and 22 inches.

Labor and Delivery

L abor is a series of continuous, progressively more intense contractions of the uterus that help the cervix to efface (thin) and dilate (open), allowing the fetus to move through the birth canal. Labor usually starts 2 weeks before or after the estimated date of delivery. No one knows exactly what triggers the onset of labor, and each pregnant woman experiences labor differently.

Some common signs of labor may include the following:

1. Bloody show. This term is used when a small amount of mucus, slightly mixed with blood, is expelled from the vagina, indicating that labor has started.

2. Contractions. Uterine muscle spasms occurring at intervals of less than 10 minutes are usually an indication that labor has begun. These contractions may become more frequent and severe as labor progresses.

3. Rupture of the amniotic sac membranes ("bag of waters"). Labor sometimes begins with the rupture of the amniotic sac and the gushing or leaking of amniotic fluid from the vagina. Women who experience this should contact their obstetrician immediately. The majority of women with ruptured membranes go into labor within 24 hours. If labor has not begun after 24 hours, the woman may be hospitalized so labor can be induced. This step is often taken to prevent infections and delivery complications. Call your doctor if you are uncertain about whether your labor has begun.

Labor and delivery are usually normal for women with epilepsy. Antiepileptic medications can be given intravenously during labor to reduce the risk of a seizure. Babies sometimes have symptoms of withdrawal from the mother's seizure medication, but these symptoms wear off after a few months and usually do not cause long-term problems.

Women in the United States who have epilepsy give birth to approximately 20,000 newborns every year. The authors have attempted to define the rate, risks, and causes of seizures during labor and delivery, because seizures during late development and delivery may seriously affect the fetus, and because primary generalized tonic-clonic (GTC) seizures may occur during labor and delivery in 1% to 2% percent of women with epilepsy.

In one study, 89 pregnant women taking AEDs for epilepsy were analyzed. Six epileptologists in the group had treated these patients. The study established data and acquired new information by telephone for 83.1% of the pregnancies and categorized the women as having primary generalized or partial epilepsy. The results showed that 78% were on monotherapy, 20% took two AEDs during pregnancy, and 2% took three AEDs during pregnancy.

Seizures during labor and delivery occurred in 4 out of 32 patients (12.5%) with primary generalized epilepsy, but in none of the 57 women with partial epilepsy. None of the 38 patients with therapeutic antiepileptic drug levels before labor and delivery had seizures, compared to 3 out of 37 (8.1%) of the subtherapeutic group. Drug levels were taken at variable times in relation to delivery, limiting their value. The levels sampled were both total and free levels; the final levels would be more helpful to determine the sufficiency of antiepileptic drug coverage.

Maintaining therapeutic antiepileptic drug levels during the last trimester may help prevent seizures during labor and delivery, especially in women with generalized epilepsy. Women with epilepsy who had subtherapeutic antiepileptic drug levels before pregnancy, and had been seizure-free, may be at risk for seizures during labor and delivery.

At the Hospital

It is important to tell the medical team who will attend the birth of your baby that you have epilepsy, including the type of seizures you have had in the past and what medication you are currently taking. It is also helpful to tell hospital staff about anything that has caused you to have a seizure in the past, such as pain, exhaustion, or heavy breathing.

When you arrive at the hospital in labor, the medical staff will perform a physical examination of your abdomen to determine the size and position of the fetus, and an examination of your cervix to ascertain how much it has dilated. The following will also be checked: blood pressure, weight, temperature, frequency and intensity of contractions, fetal heart rate, and urine and blood samples.

Intravenous fluids are sometimes given during labor to prevent dehydration, and an intravenous line (IV) may be started. The IV is a thin plastic tube that is inserted into a vein (usually in the forearm) and may also be used to administer medications.

A device may be placed on the mother's abdomen to monitor the fetal heart rate.

Pain Relief

A woman has many options for managing the discomforts that occur during labor and delivery. Normally, mothers and their obstetricians will use the method of pain relief that is safest and most effective for both mother and baby. This choice will be determined by patient and family preference and by the health of the patient and the fetus. Discuss the risks and benefits of the various methods of pain relief with your obstetrician and anesthesiologist in advance. The following methods of pain relief are often recommended:

ANALGESICS

The smallest possible dose of pain medication is given because of the potential adverse effects of these medications on the fetus. These medications easily cross the placenta to the fetus and may take a long time to clear from the baby's system after birth. Many analgesics can cause respiratory depression in mothers and babies if they are given in large amounts or repeated doses. Pethidine can set off seizures in some women and is therefore not recommended for women who have epilepsy.

ANESTHESIA

Anesthetics are medications that cause loss of sensation and are administered in different ways.

Local Block

When using this method, anesthesia is injected into the perineal area—the area between the vagina and rectum—in order to numb the area for repairing a tear or episiotomy after delivery. (An episiotomy is a surgical procedure that involves cutting the perineum during labor to enlarge the vaginal opening.)

Pudendal Block

This type of local anesthesia is injected into the vaginal area (affecting the pudendal nerve), causing complete numbness in the vaginal area without affecting the contractions of the uterus. When using this method, the woman can remain active in pushing the baby through the birth canal. The pudendal block is used for vaginal deliveries.

Epidural Anesthesia (Also Called an Epidural Block)

This type of anesthesia involves administering medications through a thin catheter that has been inserted into the space surrounding the spinal cord in the low back, causing loss of sensation of the lower body. The amount of medication may be increased or decreased as needed. This type of anesthesia is used during labor and for vaginal and cesarean deliveries. The most common complication of epidural anesthesia is low blood pressure in the mother, and most woman need to receive intravenous fluids before epidural anesthesia is given in order to avoid this potential side effect. Epidural analgesia is sometimes called a "walking" medication, because it relieves pain but does not numb the body, thereby allowing movement. Combinations of medications may be used in an epidural—part analgesic, part anesthetic. Postpartum headache may occur if the epidural needle enters the spinal canal rather than staying in the space around the canal.

Spinal Anesthesia

This type of anesthesia involves injecting a single dose of the anesthetic agent directly into the spinal cord canal. Spinal anesthesia acts very quickly, causing complete loss of sensation and loss of the ability to move the lower body. This type of anesthesia is often used for caesarean deliveries.

General Anesthesia

This type of pain relief involves administering an anesthetic that causes the woman to go to sleep. It may be used during emergency cesarean deliveries.

OTHER TYPES OF PAIN RELIEF

Other types of pain relief provide comfort and relieve stress. Many women learn special techniques in a childbirth class to help them feel more comfortable and in control during labor and birth. These include some of the following techniques:

1. Relaxation techniques. Using a progressive relaxation technique, various muscle groups are relaxed one by one in order to help detect tension and then release it

2. TENS machine (transcutaneous electrical nerve stimulator, which uses electrical impulses to stop pain signals getting to the brain).

3. Massage. Have your partner, friend, or birth coach lightly massage tense areas of your body to relieve tension.

4. Heat or cold therapy. A warm towel or a cold pack may be used to help relax tense or painful areas.

5. Imagery. This technique uses the mind to form mental pictures that can aid in relaxation.

6. Meditation and breathing techniques. Focusing on an object or task, such as breathing, helps direct the mind away from the discomforts of labor and delivery. These techniques can be learned in a class.

7. Warm showers or a bath. Warm water is an effective tool for relaxation.

8. Positioning and movement. Many women find that changing positions and movement during labor help relieve discomfort and may even speed labor along. Various positions are suggested:

   ❖ Rock in a rocking chair.

   ❖ Assume the "tailor sit" position: sit on the floor with knees bent and feet crossed (a relaxed cross-legged position). This position gives the inner thighs a good stretch and takes the pressure off the low back.

   ❖ Sit on a special "birthing ball."

   ❖ Walk or sway.

Your labor nurse or obstetrician can help you find comfortable positions that are safe for you and your baby.

Stages of Labor

The process of labor and childbirth is divided into three stages: The first stage of labor consists of an early phase, which begins with the onset of contractions and the gradual effacement (thinning out) and dilation (opening) of the cervix. The next phase of stage one is called the active phase, during which the cervix begins to dilate more rapidly, and the contractions are longer, stronger, and closer together. This is usually the time to call the doctor. The active phase ends with the transition period, during which the cervix fully dilates to 10 centimeters.

The second stage begins once you are fully dilated, and ends with the birth of the baby. This period is often referred to as the pushing stage.

The third stage begins immediately after the birth of the baby, and involves the separation and delivery of the placenta.

In some cases, labor has to be induced, a process of stimulating labor to start. Some common reasons for induction include the following:

* ❖ The mother and/or fetus are at risk.

* ❖ The pregnancy has continued too far past the due date.

* ❖ The mother has preeclampsia, eclampsia, or chronic hypertension.

* ❖ There has been a diagnosis of poor growth of the fetus.

Some common techniques of induction include inserting vaginal suppositories containing the hormone prostaglandin; administering an intravenous infusion of oxytocin or a similar drug, or artificially rupturing the amniotic sac membranes.

The process of labor and delivery takes an average of 15 hours for first-time mothers, although for many women it lasts longer than 20 hours. Subsequent deliveries average around 8 hours.

STAGE ONE, EARLY PHASE

It is often hard to tell exactly when the regular contractions of the first stage of labor begin, because they may be hard to distinguish from the irregular, inefficient Braxton Hicks contractions that usually precede them.

Labor has officially begun, however, once your contractions begin occurring at regular intervals and your cervix begins to dilate.

The contractions will gradually become stronger and more frequent, and last longer. Although the experience of labor can vary widely, a typical labor will start out with contractions coming every 10 minutes, lasting 30 seconds each, and then gradually increasing to every 5 minutes, lasting 40 to 60 seconds each.

Some women have more frequent contractions during the first phase of stage one, although they tend to be mild and last less than a minute. You may also notice a mucous discharge from the vagina that may be tinged with blood. This is perfectly normal, but if you see more than a tinge of blood, be sure to call your doctor. You should also call your doctor if your bag of water breaks, even if you are not having any contractions. The early phase ends when your cervix is approximately 3 to 5 centimeters dilated, and labor starts to accelerate. This phase can take from 12 to 14 hours, or longer, although it is often considerably shorter for subsequent babies.

Your contractions will become more regular, more intense, and more painful than the earlier Braxton Hicks contractions you may have experienced. Sometimes these contractions can be quite painful. If you are typical, however, your contractions during this phase will not require the same attention they will later in labor. You will probably be able to talk during contractions and putter around the house. You may want to take a walk or a warm bath or watch a video.

Do not become a slave to your stopwatch during early labor, because it can be stressful and exhausting. Instead, you may want to time your contractions periodically to get a sense of what is going on. In most cases, the contractions will let you know (in no uncertain terms) when it is time to take them more seriously. Meanwhile, it is important to do your best to stay rested, because you may have a long day or night ahead of you. Some women even doze off between contractions. (If you are able to sleep through them, you are probably not in true labor yet.) Also, be sure to drink plenty of fluids and urinate frequently even if you do not feel the urge, because an empty bladder leaves more room for the baby to descend.

STAGE ONE, ACTIVE PHASE

During the active phase of stage one labor, your contractions will become more frequent, longer, and stronger, and your cervix will begin dilating faster. As a general rule, once you have had regular, painful contractions (each lasting approximately 60 seconds) every 5 minutes for an hour, it is time to call your midwife or obstetrician. (The doctor may prefer to receive an early warning call; discuss this in advance.) In most cases, the frequency of contractions eventually increases to once every 2 to 3 minutes, although some women have contractions only once every 4 to 5 minutes.

The active phase of stage one labor can last up to 6 hours, or more, although it can be shorter, especially if you have previously had a vaginal delivery. Now the real work of labor begins, and you will no longer be able to talk during contractions. Breathing exercises, relaxation techniques, and a good labor coach can be helpful during this phase. Massage and gentle encouragement can also be helpful.

By now, you have probably arrived at the hospital or birth center. If you have no medical or obstetric complications, you should be able to move around. You may find that it feels good to walk, but you will probably want to stop and lean against someone or something during contractions. If you feel exhausted, sit in a rocking chair or lie in bed on your left side. This might be a good time to take a warm shower or bath if you have access to these facilities. Warm water can help ease the pain of labor, and women sometimes progress quite rapidly with the relaxation that water provides.

You may want to ask for general or regional analgesia if you are having difficulty coping with pain during the second phase of stage-one labor. You will still feel contractions with systemic pain relief (usually delivered by IV or injection), but to a lesser extent. The medication might make you feel drowsy or dizzy, and you will not be allowed to walk around after receiving it. Generally, regional anesthesia (such as an epidural or spinal, or both) will provide more complete pain relief, although you might continue to feel some pressure if the baby is low in your pelvis.

The last part of the active phase of stage one is called transition, because it marks the transition to the second stage of labor. Contractions are usually very strong during transition, coming approximately every 2½ to 3 minutes, and lasting a minute or longer. The cervix continues to dilate until it reaches the full 10 centimeters.

Transition can last anywhere from a few minutes to a few hours. It is much more likely to be rapid if you have previously had a vaginal delivery. This is the most intense phase of labor, with contractions coming hard and fast, and symptoms that may include shaking, shivering, and nausea. Some women who have been coping well up to this point may begin to lose control during transition. They might reject those around them, but clearly have trouble being left alone. Some women who have previously expressed the desire for a drug-free birth may begin to lose faith in their ability to deliver the baby without medication. This is the time when you will need plenty of encouragement. If you have made it this far without medication, you can usually be coached through transition—one contraction at a time—with reminders that you are doing a great job and the baby will arrive soon.

By the end of the first stage of labor, when the cervix reaches full dilation, the baby has usually descended somewhat into the pelvic area. You might begin to feel rectal pressure, as if you have to move your bowels. Some women begin to bear down spontaneously, and may even start making some deep grunting sounds. There is often a lot more bloody discharge. You may also feel nauseated, or even vomit, as you make the transition to the second stage of labor.

If you have an epidural, you will feel varying amounts of pressure, depending on the type and amount of medication. If you want to be a more active participant in the second stage of labor, ask to have the dose reduced at the end of the first stage of labor.

STAGE TWO

Once your cervix is fully dilated, the work of the second stage begins: the descent and ultimate birth of your baby. This stage can last anywhere from a few minutes to hours. The average duration of the second stage is close to an hour for a first baby (or longer if you have an epidural), and 20 minutes if you have previously had a vaginal delivery.

Your contractions may be a little further apart during the second stage than during transition, giving you the chance for a much-needed and well-deserved rest between them. Some women feel an involuntary urge to push early in the second stage, whereas others do not have this sensation until the baby is lower down. Depending on your wishes, your particular situation, and the practice patterns of your doctor or midwife, you may be coached to push with each contraction in an effort to speed up the baby's descent. Alternatively, you might take it more slowly and wait until you spontaneously feel the urge to push. You will need explicit coaching to help you to push effectively if you have an epidural.

Although it can be difficult and exhausting, many women find the work of the second stage to be extremely gratifying. Some women find the intense sensation of pressure while pushing to be very uncomfortable and even frightening, but many laboring mothers find that working with the contractions and being an active participant helps to dull the pain of contractions.

It is important to pay attention to the signals your body gives you during the second stage of labor. Try different positions for pushing until you find one that feels right and is effective. Squatting or sitting works well for some women, but not for all women. If you have back labor (where the baby is positioned face up and the back of its head is against your spine), you might find that pushing while you are on all fours is more comfortable and effective. Pushing while lying on your left side often works quite well, and can allow you to rest between contractions. It is not unusual to use a variety of different positions during the second stage.

With each contraction, the force of your uterus—combined with the force of your abdominal muscles if you are actively pushing—exerts pressure on the baby, which moves the baby down through the birth canal. The baby's head will recede slightly when a contraction is over and your uterus relaxes. In this way, labor progresses in a "two steps forward, one step back" manner.

At some point, the perineum (the skin between the vagina and the anus) will begin to bulge with each push, and the baby's scalp will become visible. You can ask for a mirror to get your first glimpse of the baby, or you may simply reach down and touch the top of the baby's head.

The urge to push soon becomes quite compelling. The baby's head becomes more and more visible with each contraction. The pressure of the head on the perineum may be very intense, and you may experience an unpleasant burning sensation as the tissue begins to stretch. You may be asked to push more gently (or not to push at all), so that the head can gradually stretch out your vagina and perineum. A slow, controlled birth is essential in preventing the skin from tearing. The urge to push can become so overwhelming, however, that you may be coached to blow or pant to help you slow down.

The baby's head continues to advance with each push until it crowns. This term describes the moment when the widest part of the baby's head is finally visible. The excitement in the room will be palpable as the baby's face begins to appear: the forehead, nose, mouth, and, finally, the chin. It is a moment of unparalleled beauty.

You will be coached to pant after the head is delivered, while your midwife or doctor suctions the baby's mouth and nose, and feels around the baby's neck for the umbilical cord. (No need to worry. If the cord is around the baby's neck, it will either be slipped over the baby's head or, if necessary, doubly clamped and cut.) The baby's head will then be turned to the side, and the shoulders will rotate inside the pelvis in order to get into position for the completion of the birth. With the next contraction, you will be coached to push as the shoulders are delivered, one at a time, followed by the rest of the body.

Tell your doctor ahead of time that you want your baby to be lifted onto your bare abdomen as soon as he or she is born—if there have been no complications during the birth—so that you can touch, kiss, and simply marvel at your child. The skin-to-skin contact will keep your baby warm, and the bonding between you and the baby can begin immediately.

You have received the greatest gift: a baby! It is a special moment that will stay with you and your family forever. You may cry or shout; you may feel scared, full of pride, or worried about whether you will be a good mother. You will be excited and relieved. Although you are exhausted, you are also likely to feel a huge burst of energy, and any thoughts of immediate sleep will vanish.

STAGE THREE

The mild contractions of the third stage of labor generally begin 3 to 5 minutes after the arrival of the baby. The placenta is delivered during this stage. It may take only a few minutes or last up to 30 minutes or so. On average, you can expect it to take approximately 5 to 10 minutes.

The first few contractions usually separate the placenta from the uterine wall. When the doctor sees signs of separation, he may ask you to push gently to help expel the placenta. This usually requires one short push that is not difficult or painful. Your uterus should contract and become quite firm after delivery of the placenta. You will be able to feel the top of your uterus in your abdomen at approximately the level of your navel. Your doctor, and later a nurse, will periodically check to see that it remains firm. A well-contracted uterus is necessary to prevent continued bleeding from the former site of placental attachment. Nursing the baby will trigger your body to release oxytocin, a hormone that not only acts on the breast to release milk, but also helps to keep the uterus well contracted. If you are not nursing, or if you are bleeding excessively, you may be given medication to help your uterus contract.

During the final stage of labor, you may be oblivious to whatever else is going on around you, because you are focused on the baby. If this is your first baby, you may feel a few contractions after you have delivered the placenta. You may continue to feel contractions intermittently for the next day or two if you have previously had a baby. These contractions are known as afterbirth pains. They are similar to strong menstrual cramps. Ask the doctor for pain medication if necessary. You may also get a case of the chills or feel shaky after the birth. This is perfectly normal and will not last long. Ask the nurse for a warm blanket.

The doctor will examine the placenta to make sure it is intact, and check you thoroughly to see if you have any tears or an episiotomy that need to be sutured. You may be given an injection of a local anesthetic before being sutured. Hold your newborn while you are getting sutured—it can be a great distraction. If you feel too shaky, however, ask your partner to sit by your side and hold the baby.

If you had an epidural during labor, the anesthesiologist or nurse anesthetist will remove the catheter from your back. (This takes only a second and does not hurt.) Unless your baby is in need of special care, be sure to insist on some quiet time together. The eye drops, vitamin K, and footprints can wait—you and your partner will want to share this special time with each other as you get acquainted with your new baby.

Recovery

Even an uncomplicated pregnancy that culminates in a relatively easy birth is an emotionally and physically exhausting experience. If your labor was longer or more difficult than you expected, or if you experienced complications, you may feel particularly worn out—not to mention confused and anxious about what to expect next.

You may also have some questions about what happened during the birth, and why. You may be wondering about future pregnancies, and how your labor experience may affect your health. Be sure to communicate your concerns to your doctor. Even if the doctor explained everything during the delivery, you might not remember what was said. Ask your doctor again, when you are able to concentrate and retain the information.

Tips for a fast, easy recovery:

❖ Sleep when the baby sleeps.

❖ Eat nutritious food.

❖ Drink sufficient fluids.

❖ Ask for and accept all offers for help with cooking, cleaning, childcare, or whatever else friends and family offer.

If you lost a lot of blood, became dehydrated during labor, or are anemic after childbirth, it may take you a few extra days or weeks before you start feeling normal again. If no one offers to pitch in during the early days, or if you live far from family, consider hiring a nanny. The nanny can help with childcare, housekeeping, cooking, and whatever else you need once you are home so you can rest and bond with your newborn.

After 9 Delivery

Treatment for mothers with epilepsy does not stop after the birth of the baby. It is important to see your neurologist about 4 weeks after the birth in order to check your antiepilepsy drug levels. Careful monitoring of AED levels should be performed throughout pregnancy and after delivery. Continued medication after pregnancy is especially important, because babies are totally dependent upon their mothers for care.

Mothers of newborns are often focused entirely on their babies, but they also need to take care of themselves. The desire to be a good mother is admirable, but unless you are mentally, physically, and spiritually healthy you will not able to care for your child adequately. Health is determined by personal responsibility. New mothers need to eat wholesome foods that nourish the body, mind, and spirit, especially if they are breast-feeding. Daily exercise is also very important. Exercise balances energy, strengthens the body, calms the mind, and increases confidence. Be sure to include relaxing activities in your daily schedule as well.

Stacey Chillemi's Experience

After the birth of my children, I would always try to take a leisurely bath after my husband came home, so that he could watch the children. I would listen to music that I enjoyed and burn incense. Afterward, I would feel relaxed and be more focused, and better able to care for the new baby.

Eat a healthy breakfast and go for a walk—alone or with the baby in a stroller or backpack. Maintain good posture, breathe evenly and deeply, and wear comfortable shoes. Walking is a good form of exercise for any age or fitness level, and it brings as many benefits as a high-intensity workout. It takes time to recuperate after childbirth, so start slowly.

In addition to the benefits outlined in chapter 6, walking on a regular basis

❖ improves circulation,

❖ lowers blood pressure,

❖ strengthens the heart,

❖ nourishes the immune system,

❖ relieves backaches,

❖ increases energy,

❖ helps maintain strong bones,

❖ increases concentration,

❖ decreases stress levels and anxiety, and

❖ helps a new mother to lose excess weight after pregnancy (15 to 20 pounds for most women).

Happiness is the enriching quality of embracing life with an open heart, and it expands when you have a new baby to care for and love. Remember, your health and happiness depend more on what you do for yourself than on what others do for you. Give back to yourself, and your body, mind, and spirit will be healthy.

Childcare

The risk of seizure while attending to a newborn is significant enough for most parents who are epileptic to consider alternative ways of care. Having epilepsy may not interfere with childcare if seizures are well controlled. There are certain risks in different activities, however, if seizures are not well controlled. The nature of these risks depends on the type of seizures and the activity. Seizures in which the person becomes confused or unaware of his or her behavior or loses consciousness may pose the same risk as tonic-clonic seizures.

If you have seizures that are sudden and unpredictable, it may be a useful precaution to dress, change, and feed the baby while sitting on the floor. Lean against a wall to avoid falling onto the child if you have a seizure. You can also surround yourself with cushions and beanbags when you are holding the baby.

If there is no one available to assist with bathing, sponging the baby down on a changing mat on the floor is safer than bathing the baby in a tub of water.

The following suggestions can also protect the baby or toddler:

1. Carry the baby up and down the stairs in a padded carrycot.

2. Fit the baby's pram with a deadlock so that it will stay in place even if you let go of it.

3. During feeding, use a high chair for your baby that is low to the ground because this type of chair is less likely to tip over in the event of a seizure.

4. Use safety gates to section off high-risk areas in the home.

5. Always use a safety harness when the baby is in a pram or stroller.

6. Fireguards, playpens, and stair gates will protect your toddler from dangers in the home should you have a seizure and be unable to supervise the child.

7. Consider attaching toddler reins to your wrist until your child understands the importance of staying near you in the event you have a seizure.

8. Store medications in childproof containers safely out of reach at all times.

9. Use precautionary guards on stoves and cookers.

10. Install protective childproof latches on all cabinets at the child's level.

Caring for a new baby is tiring, especially if the baby wakes often during the night. Lack of sleep may trigger seizures, so a daytime nap may be helpful for you as well as the baby. Perhaps another family member can take over some of the feedings using your expressed breast milk.

As the child gets older, it is important to discuss your seizures and medication with the child. Storybooks are available that may help you explain epilepsy to your children. Teaching the child about what to do if a parent has a seizure can be done surprisingly early on. Young children may be able to stay with the parent during a seizure, and when they get a little older, they may be able to get help if a panic alarm is available. They can also be taught to call 911. Children learn by example from the rest of the family, and if seizures are dealt with confidently, they will not be overwhelmed if a seizure occurs. Comforting the child after a parent's seizure can ease any feelings of fear they may have.

Let your family and friends know if you need help in caring for your new baby or toddler. You can also contact local community services, including those specializing in services for people with epilepsy.

Breast-Feeding

Breast-feeding is beneficial for all women and their babies, and women who take medicine for epilepsy can breast-feed safely. If the mother was taking AEDs while she was pregnant, the amount of medication consumed by the baby through breast milk is significantly lower than the amount the baby was exposed to in the womb. Therefore, the benefits of breast-feeding usually outweigh the risks. Some AEDs have side effects, however. Phenobarbital or primidone may result in the baby's being overly sleepy, and if you must take these AEDs, you may have to bottle-feed instead. If your baby's pediatrician and your neurologist work together, however, you will probably be able to continue to breast-feed your baby by adjusting your AEDs.

Learn as much as you can in advance about breast-feeding. There are several ways to conduct your own research:

❖ Reading (including new prescription patient information brochures)

❖ Watching videos

❖ Talking to other women who have breast-fed

❖ Attending a class at a hospital or other health organization

❖ Discussing your questions and concerns with your neurologist and obstetrician

❖ Consulting prenatal instructors or a lactation consultant at your local hospital

❖ Searching the Internet

Get approval from your doctor for all medications that you take during pregnancy and after delivery, including nonprescription medications. Doctors often caution mothers who have been treated with certain medications about the tendency of these AEDs to remain at high levels in breast milk.

Research has shown that it is good for women to breast-feed their babies for a least a few weeks. This will naturally wean the baby from the medication they were exposed to throughout the pregnancy. Most women will be able to produce adequate milk to feed their babies, and they will also be able to keep nursing if they decide to go back to work.

There are significant differences between human milk and infant formula. Human milk provides all the protein, sugar, fat, and vitamins your baby needs to be healthy, but it also has special benefits that formula does not. Because of the protective substances in human milk, breast-fed children are less likely to have ear infections, allergies, vomiting, diarrhea, pneumonia, wheezing, bronchitis, and meningitis.

There are other reasons why human milk is good for babies. Studies have shown that breast-feeding may help protect against sudden infant death syndrome (SIDS), and it is easier for babies to digest. Breast milk does not need to be prepared, it saves money, and is always available.

Breast-feeding is good for mothers because it burns additional calories, helps maintain strong bones, and reduces the risk of ovarian and breast cancer. It also delays the return of your menstrual period, which may help extend the time between pregnancies, and helps the uterus return to its normal size.

The longer you breast-feed, the greater the benefits will be to you and your baby, and the longer these benefits will last. The World Health Organization and many other experts encourage women to breast-feed for one year or longer because human milk provides the best nutrition and protection against infections. It also promotes maternal–child bonding.

It is helpful to have the support of your family and friends if you are going to breast-feed. The baby's father cannot experience breast-feeding in the same way you do, but he can share many other special, personal moments with the baby. Older brothers and sisters can help by holding the baby, changing diapers, and playing with the baby.

Let your neurologist and obstetrician know in advance about your plans to breast-feed. It is best to start breast-feeding within the first hour after birth if possible. You and your baby should stay together as much as possible while you are in the hospital. Having your baby in the same room with you during your stay at the hospital has been shown to help make breast-feeding more successful.

Your body automatically starts to get ready for breast-feeding when you become pregnant and is able to produce milk during the fourth or fifth month of pregnancy. The first milk produced after the birth is called colostrum, and it contains all of the nutrients your baby needs. Colostrum is thick and yellowish or orange in color. Your body will produce colostrum for several days after delivery until the developed milk "comes in." The milk gradually becomes thinner and whiter, and begins to adapt to the baby's needs. One of the most amazing qualities about human milk is that it changes in response to the changing needs of the growing baby.

During pregnancy, your body increases the manufacture of a hormone called prolactin, which stimulates the cells in your breasts to make milk. The amount of prolactin also increases when you nurse your baby. It does not matter how large your breasts are; size is not an issue in milk production—the act of nursing controls milk production. The more you nurse, the more milk your body will produce.

You do not have to care for your nipples or breasts in any special way during pregnancy, but make sure your bras provide enough support. Purchase nursing bras that allow room for breast growth. Soap, lotion, or alcohol may be irritating to your breasts and should not be used. Wash your breasts with warm water only. Ask your obstetrician to examine your breasts and nipples periodically during pregnancy.

A few women have nipples that are drawn inward, or inverted. The baby may not be able to grasp the areola properly if the mother has inverted nipples. This condition is not common and usually improves on its own during pregnancy as the breasts get larger. Inverted nipples can be treated late in pregnancy, or soon after the baby is born if they do not improve naturally.

The baby's first feeding can take place within 30 minutes to an hour after delivery. The protection against infection that human milk provides is vital immediately after birth. Your milk will also give the baby nutrients to prevent low blood sugar. This early taste of breast milk will stimulate the baby to continue nursing.

Positions for Breast-Feeding

If you had a vaginal delivery, you can nurse in bed by lying on your side with the baby facing you. You can also nurse in a chair by cradling the baby, holding the baby's head in the crook of your arm. Firmly support the baby's back and buttocks. Make sure the baby's entire body is facing your body, not the ceiling.

If you delivered your baby by cesarean section, you can breast-feed sitting up, using one or two extra pillows to support the baby. This will help you avoid placing the baby against your abdominal incision. You can also lie down on your side with your baby facing you.

Another position for nursing mothers with a cesarean section is the "football hold." To use this position, hold the baby's legs and body under your arm, with your hand at the base of its head and neck (imagine holding a football). Place your fingers below your breast. Let the baby latch on while pulling the baby in close, holding the baby's head with its nose and chin touching your breast. Keep your baby's body flexed at the hip with its legs tucked under your arm. The football hold is also a good position to use when

❖ you need more visibility in getting your baby to latch on;

❖ your breasts are large;

❖ you are nursing a small baby, especially if premature;

❖ the baby tends to slide down your areola onto your nipple;

❖ the baby is fussy, restless, and has difficulty latching on;

❖ the baby is sleepy (sitting upright may encourage the baby to remain alert for a longer period of time);

❖ you have inverted nipples.

Always take the time to make yourself comfortable. Try sitting on the floor surrounded by cushions and leaning against the wall when feeding the baby in order to reduce the risk of injury if you should have a seizure during nursing.

Latching On

Touching your breast to the center of the baby's lips will stimulate the baby to open his mouth wide. This is called the rooting reflex. Pull the baby straightforward onto the nipple and areola. The baby is correctly positioned, or latched on, when your nipple and much of the areola are pulled well into the baby's mouth. Your baby's lips and gums should be around the areola, not on the nipple. This is why it is important for the baby's mouth to be open wide.

You can help your baby latch on by holding the breast with your free hand. Place your fingers under the breast, and rest your thumb lightly on top (behind the areola). Make sure the baby is properly lined up at your breast and that your fingers are well back from the areola so they do not get in the way.

There will be a tugging feeling when you first begin to nurse. If the latch on hurts, pinches, or produces pain, it may be incorrect. Break the latch on by slipping your finger into the corner of the baby's mouth, then reposition, and try again. This may take several tries. Breast-feeding should not be painful. Correct latching is important because it improves the flow of milk, prevents sore nipples, keeps the baby happy, stimulates a good milk supply, and helps prevent overly full (bloated) breasts.

Talk with your pediatrician or a lactation specialist if you are having difficulties with latching on, or if you have pain while breast-feeding. Babies use their lips, gums, and tongues to get the milk to flow from the breast. This is known as suckling. Simply sucking on the nipple will not draw milk and may hurt the nipple. Listen for gulping sounds so you will know for certain that the baby is actually swallowing the milk. Also watch for slow, steady jaw movements.

Most babies will nurse energetically if they are hungry and positioned correctly. For the first few weeks after birth, until breast-feeding is well established, breast-feeding newborns should not be given any supplements such as water, sugar water, or formula unless there is a medical reason for it. A baby who is breast-feeding regularly and effectively will get all the necessary water and nutrients from nursing. Some authorities believe that introducing a bottle or using a pacifier may cause nipple confusion and interfere with the establishment of breast-feeding. Others disagree, and feel that nonnutritive sucking does not interfere with breast-feeding.

The Let-Down Reflex

The body produces oxytocin, which causes muscles within the breasts to contract, pressing the milk down the milk ducts toward the nipples. This process is called the let-down reflex; it occurs each time you nurse your baby. It may take a few minutes the first few times you nurse. Afterward, let-down will occur much more quickly, usually within a few seconds. The signs of let-down are different for each woman. Sometimes, you may feel a brief itch, shiver, or even slight pain in your breast when your baby begins to nurse. Milk may even start dripping from the breast that is not being suckled.

You may feel strong cramping in your uterus when your milk lets down, because oxytocin also causes the muscles of the uterus to contract. In this way, nursing helps your uterus return to its normal size. This type of cramping is completely normal and is actually a sign of successful nursing. The cramping should go away in a week or so.

Try these tips to encourage the let-down process:

1. Sit in a comfortable chair with good support for your arms and back. A rocking chair works well.

2. Make sure your baby is in the proper position on your breast. Correct positioning is one of the most important factors in successful breast-feeding.

3. Listen to soothing music and sip a nutritious drink during feedings.

The following can interfere with let-down and affect the content of breast milk. They are not good for you and your baby:

1. Smoking. Do not smoke while you are breast-feeding or around children. Secondhand smoke is dangerous to all children, but especially to newborns, because it increases the risk of SIDS.

2. Drinking alcohol. Avoid drinking alcohol while you are nursing, because it can pass through your milk to your baby and cause fetal alcohol syndrome.

3. Illegal drugs. All illegal drugs should be avoided.

4. Birth control pills. This form of birth control may affect milk production, but the effects vary from woman to woman and with the type of pill. Discuss this with your doctor.

Wear nursing bras and clothes that are easy to undo. Nursing bras have front closing flaps that come down to expose your nipple and part of your breast. If your household is very busy, set aside a quiet place ahead of time where you will not be disturbed during feedings. Sometimes just thinking about your baby helps let-down occur.

Breast Care

By the third or fourth day of breast-feeding, your milk will become thicker and begin to resemble skim milk. Your breasts will also become firm. If your nipples leak, use a nursing pad or clean folded handkerchief squares inside your bra to catch the leaking milk. Be sure to change these often. Do not use plastic-lined pads because they prevent air from circulating around your nipples. Between feedings, gently pat your nipples dry. This helps prevent irritation. You may also want to apply a little expressed colostrum, human milk, or medical-grade modified lanolin on your nipples to prevent dryness.

You may develop cracked or sore nipples if your baby is not positioned properly or does not latch on correctly. Reposition the baby frequently to prevent these problems, and make sure the baby's lips and gums are on the areola, not on the nipple.

Breast-Feeding Patterns

Breast-fed babies tend to feed more often than formula-fed babies do, usually 8 to 12 times per day. The main reason for this is that their stomachs empty quickly because human milk is so easy to digest.

At first, your newborn will probably nurse every couple of hours, day or night. By the end of the first month, your baby may start sleeping longer at night. Let your baby feed on demand—that is, whenever the baby is hungry. Watch for signals from the baby rather than the clock. The baby will let you know he or she is hungry by crying, snuggling against your breast, making rooting reflex or sucking motions, or putting its hand to its mouth.

It is best not to wait until your baby is overly hungry before you breast-feed. Some newborns can be sleepy and hard to wake. Do not let your baby sleep through feeding times until your milk supply has been well developed, usually about 2 to 3 weeks. If the baby is not demanding to be fed, wake the baby if 3 to 4 hours have passed since the last feeding. Call your pediatrician if this pattern continues.

Some infants nurse for only 10 minutes on one breast, but it is quite common for others to stay on one side for much longer. Some feedings may be longer than others, depending on your baby's schedule and the time of day. Some babies may be nursing even though they appear to be sleeping. If the baby has fallen asleep at your breast, or if you need to stop nursing before the baby is finished, gently break the suction with your finger by slipping a finger into the baby's mouth. Never pull the baby off the breast without first releasing the suction.

Alternate which breast you offer first. You may want to keep a safety pin or short ribbon on your bra strap to help you remember on which breast your baby last nursed. Although you should try to breast-feed evenly on both sides, your baby may prefer one side to the other, and nurse much longer on that side. In this case, your body may adapt milk production to your baby's preferences. Remember, nursing controls how much milk your breasts produce, and it is important to let your baby nurse on both sides so that each breast gets equal stimulation.

You will soon get to know your baby's feeding pattern. Each baby has a particular style of nursing, some slower, some faster. Learning the baby's pattern will make it easier to determine when the baby is hungry and when the baby has had enough to eat.

Engorgement

Nursing on demand not only ensures that the baby's hunger will be satisfied, but it also helps prevent engorgement, which can occur when your breasts become too full of milk. A little engorgement is normal, but excessive engorgement can be uncomfortable or painful. If your breasts become engorged, try the following:

❖ Squeeze out some milk before you breast-feed, either manually or with a breast pump.

❖ Soak a cloth in warm water and apply it to your breasts, or you can take a warm shower before feeding the baby. Warmth may not help severe inflammation, however. In this case, you may want to use cold compresses as you express milk. Ice packs used between feedings can relieve discomfort and reduce swelling.

❖ Feed your baby in more than one position. Try sitting up, then lying down.

❖ Gently massage your breasts from under the arm and down toward the nipple. This will help reduce soreness and ease milk flow.

❖ Do not take any medications without approval from your doctor. Acetaminophen (Tylenol) may be taken for occasional pain relief.

❖ It is important to continue breast-feeding. Engorgement is a temporary condition that is quickly relieved by effective milk removal.

❖ Your breasts will become soft again once the engorgement passes. This is normal.

You can express milk manually with your hands or with a breast pump. Breast pumps are used to ease engorgement and to collect milk when you are away from your baby (for example, if you are ill or at work). Pumping enables you to continue to breast-feed by keeping your milk production stimulated. Your body will stop producing milk if the milk is not emptied from the breast regularly.

To express milk manually:

1. Make sure your hands are clean; wash them well with soap and water.

2. Put a clean cup or container under your breast.

3. Massage the breasts gently toward the nipples.

4. Place your thumb about 1 inch back from the tip of the nipple and your first finger opposite.

5. Press back toward your chest, gently press the areola between the thumb and finger, and release with a rhythmic motion until the milk flows or squirts out.

6. Rotate your thumb and finger around the areola to get milk from several positions.

7. Transfer the milk into clean, covered containers for storage in the refrigerator or freezer for possible later feedings.

8. Always label the container and date it.

Some women prefer to use hand expression because it can be done silently and does not require special equipment. Other women may find it easier and faster to express milk with a breast pump. These pumps are manual, battery-operated, or electric. You can find manual pumps in most pharmacies and baby stores. (Do not buy the type of pump that resembles a bicycle horn; it cannot be cleaned properly and the milk may become contaminated.)

The preferred pump has two cylinders, one inside the other, attached to a rigid funnel that fits over the breast. As you slide the outer cylinder up and down, negative pressure is created over the nipple area. This causes milk to collect in the bottom of the cylinder. This collecting cylinder can be used with a special nipple to feed your baby without transferring the milk. The entire pump can be cleaned in the dishwasher, or by hand with soap and hot water.

Some hand pumps have a handle for squeezing, which creates negative pressure and draws the milk into a bottle. They may have a soft, pliable flange that fits around the nipple and areola, producing a milking action while pumping.

For most women, electric pumps stimulate the breast more effectively than manual expression or hand pumps. They are used mainly to keep up milk production when a mother is not able to breast-feed for several days or more. These pumps are easier and more efficient than hand pumps, but they are much more expensive. You may be able to save money by renting an electric pump from your hospital or a medical supply store.

When shopping for an electric pump to buy or rent, make sure that it creates a milking action and is not simply a sucking device. Pumps that express milk from both breasts at the same time increase the amount of milk collected and save time. No matter which type of pump you choose, make sure that all the parts of it that come into contact with your skin or milk can be removed and cleaned. Otherwise, the pump will become a breeding ground for bacteria, and the milk will not be safe for your baby.

Spitting Up

Spitting up is a common reaction during or after feeding, and some infants just spit up more easily than others do. There is usually no need to be concerned when your baby spits up. Unlike formula-fed babies, human milk does not smell bad or stain clothing or linen.

Try the following suggestions if your baby spits up:

❖ Make sure each feeding is calm, quiet, and relaxing.

❖ Avoid interruptions, sudden noises, bright lights, and other distractions.

❖ Burp your baby at least twice during the feeding.

❖ Hold your baby upright during feedings.

❖ Put your baby in an upright position right after a feeding.

❖ Do not shove or play vigorously with your baby right after a feeding.

❖ If the baby repeatedly vomits, especially in a forceful manner, call your pediatrician right away.

❖ Most babies hiccup from time to time during feedings; continue to nurse your baby and the hiccups will stop.

Infant Nutrition

There are several ways you can tell whether your baby is getting enough milk. One is by the number of wet diapers produced daily. Make sure your baby has at least six wet diapers per day with pale yellow urine, not deep yellow or orange, beginning around the third or fourth day of life. Your infant should also have several small bowel movements daily (there may be one after every feeding during the first few weeks). Your infant should have at least two stools per day during the first week of life. From about 1 to 4 weeks old, bowel movements should increase to at least 5 per day. As your baby gets older, bowel movements may occur less often, and may even skip a number of days. Your baby's stools should be loose and yellowish in color, not white or clay-colored. The bowel movements of breast-fed babies usually smell somewhat sweeter than the stools of formula-fed babies.

Feeding patterns are also an important sign that the baby is nursing enough. A newborn may nurse every $1^1/2$ to 3 hours around the clock. If your baby sleeps longer than 4 hours at a time during the first 2 weeks, wake the baby for a feeding.

The baby should steadily gain weight after the first week of life. During the first week, some infants lose several ounces of weight, but they should be back up to their birth weight by the end of the second week. Your pediatrician will weigh your baby at each visit. Keep in mind that the baby may breast-feed more often during growth spurts.

Most breast-fed babies do not need any water, vitamins, or iron to supplement breast milk for at least the first 6 months. Human milk provides all the fluids and nutrients a baby needs to be healthy. By about 6 months of age, however, you should start to introduce your infant to baby foods that contain iron. Your pediatrician may prescribe vitamin D.

The American Academy of Pediatrics and the American Academy of Pediatric Dentistry recommend that breast-fed infants (as well as bottle-fed infants) not receive fluoride supplements during the first 6 months of life. After 6 months of age, check with your pediatrician to see if you need to give your baby fluoride.

Breast-Feeding Difficulties

If your baby cannot nurse or if you are having troubles with breast-feeding, it is important that you call your doctor as soon as possible. Refusal to breast-feed may be a sign of sickness that needs prompt attention.

Try to avoid caffeine while you are breast-feeding, or at least reduce your intake. Caffeine tends to build up in babies because their bodies cannot get rid of it very easily. A morning cup of coffee is not likely to harm your baby, but too much caffeine can cause problems such as poor sleeping, nervousness, irritability, and poor feeding. Try using decaffeinated coffee and tea, and avoid colas and other carbonated drinks that have added caffeine.

Sometimes breast-feeding babies react to certain foods eaten by their mothers. You may notice after you eat spicy or gas-producing foods that your baby cries, fusses, or nurses more often. Babies with colic often have similar symptoms. The best way to tell the difference between a food reaction and colic is by how long the symptoms last. The symptoms of a reaction to food are usually short-lived, lasting less than 24 hours. Symptoms caused by colic occur daily, and often last for days or weeks at a time. If your baby gets symptoms every time you eat a certain type of food, stop eating that particular item.

In rare instances, your breast-fed infant may be allergic to the cow's milk in your diet. Symptoms can appear anywhere from a few minutes to a few hours after the baby breast-feeds and may include diarrhea, rash, fussiness, and gas. If you suspect this possibility, cut out all dairy products from your diet for 2 weeks. Then, reintroduce each dairy product into your diet, one by one, to see whether the baby has a reaction.

BREAST-FEEDING DURING ILLNESS

Many parents are concerned that breast-feeding has to stop if the mother gets ill. During most illnesses, including colds, flu, bacterial infections, and even surgical conditions, breast-feeding can and should continue. By the time you show symptoms of an illness, your baby has already been exposed to it. The best thing to do is to keep breast-feeding, because you have already started to produce antibodies. The baby will receive these antibodies through your milk, preventing infection of the baby. If you stop breast-feeding when cold or flu symptoms first appear, you actually reduce your baby's protection and increase the chance of the baby's getting sick. If you are unable to breast-feed your baby while you are ill, keep up your milk supply by expressing milk for your baby either by hand or using a pump. The milk can then be fed to the baby.

You will usually need to stop breast-feeding only for a short period of time, even with serious illnesses. There are several infectious diseases, however, that can be transmitted by breast milk to babies, including HIV and untreated tuberculosis. Mothers with HIV are advised not to breast-feed. Similarly, mothers with tuberculosis should not breast-feed.

Mothers with hepatitis B can breast-feed their infants if the infant receives the hepatitis B vaccine during the first few days after birth. There is no evidence that hepatitis C is transmitted by breast-feeding. Mothers with chronic hepatitis C are often advised that they can nurse their infants, but they should discuss this with their physician. Other types of infections need to be evaluated by the obstetrician and pediatrician, but nearly all are likely to be safe for breast-feeding.

MASTITIS

Mastitis is an infection of the breast that causes swelling, burning, redness, and pain. It is usually caused by bacteria that enter the breast via damaged nipples. Mastitis usually occurs in just one breast, and may cause a nursing mother to feel feverish and ill. If you have any of these symptoms, let your doctor know at once so that you can start treatment. Mastitis usually develops in nursing mothers about a month after childbirth. Sometimes there is a discharge of pus. Rest and good nutrition will help you get back your energy.

Frequent nursing will help drain your breasts and prevent the infection from spreading, so it is important to keep the milk flowing in the infected breast. If it is too painful to have your baby nurse on the infected breast, open up both sides of your bra and let the milk flow from that breast onto a towel or absorbent cloth. This relieves the pressure as you feed the baby on the opposite side. Pumping the affected side may also be necessary.

IMPLANTS AND PLASTIC SURGERY

There is still some question about whether it is safe to breast-feed if you have silicone breast implants, but there is no conclusive evidence that infants are harmed. The surgery for breast implants usually does not interfere with milk ducts or the nipples unless the incision was made around the edge of the areola. This surgery should not prevent successful nursing.

Plastic surgery to reduce the size of breasts may interfere with breast-feeding, especially if the nipples were transplanted. If you have had plastic surgery on your breasts, it may be that the only way to find out whether or not you can productively breast-feed is by trying.

SPECIAL CIRCUMSTANCES

Premature and Seriously Ill Babies

Many premature and seriously ill babies are unable to breast-feed. If your baby is not able to nurse following delivery, collect your milk and feed the baby by tube or bottle. Express your milk by hand or by using an electric pump at the times when the baby would normally nurse, so that your body becomes used to the schedule, usually about eight times per day. Human milk has been shown to be very beneficial to premature and sick newborns by helping growth and preventing many diseases.

Multiple Births

It is possible to breast-feed twins at the same time by nursing one baby at each breast. You can hold one baby at each side using the football hold (described earlier), or you can cradle them both in front of you with their bodies crossing each other as they would have been in utero. Alternate the breast each baby uses at each feeding, or at least once a day. If this is too difficult, or if you are not producing enough milk, you may supplement feedings with formula.

It is also possible to breast-feed triplets, but most mothers supplement feedings with formula. Nurse two of the babies at a time and give formula to the third. At the next feeding, give the formula to a different baby. It is important that all three babies have an equal opportunity to breast-feed.

Returning to Work

Human milk has the same important benefits for older babies as it does for infants. Just because you are returning to work does not mean you have to stop breast-feeding. Knowing that you will be able to provide milk for your baby while you are away will help ease your transition back to work.

Working women can manage breast-feeding in the following ways:

❖ Extend maternity leave so there will be more time for breast-feeding to become well established.

❖ Nurse your baby once or more during the workday if the baby is in a childcare facility at your workplace or nearby.

❖ Consider working at home.

❖ Work part-time, and nurse before going to work and upon returning home.

❖ Express milk every 3 to 4 hours while you are at work for your baby to drink later from a bottle or cup.

❖ Breast-feed when you are with your baby. When you are away, the baby will receive formula or solids (if approximately 6 months of age).

❖ Be sure to select a childcare provider or center that supports breast-feeding, and can safely handle the milk and feedings per your instructions. Also, engage the support of your boss, human resources staff, occupational nurse, and coworkers. Assure them that pumping milk will not interfere with your work duties.

If possible, go back to work on a part-time or flexible schedule at first. This can help you and your baby adjust to the new routine. If this is not possible, go back to work in the middle of the week to make it easier for you and your baby to adjust.

You will need to find a quiet, private place at work to express milk, such as an unoccupied office, the bathroom, or wherever privacy can be assured. Expressing milk takes 15 to 30 minutes. You will need access to soap and water to wash your hands before expressing. You will also need a refrigerator or a small cooler and ice packs to keep the milk cold until you take it home.

Follow these safe storage and preparation tips to keep your expressed milk healthy for your baby.

1. Always wash your hands before expressing or handling your milk.

2. Be sure to use only clean containers to store expressed milk. Use screw cap bottles, hard plastic cups with tight caps, or special heavy nursery bags to store milk. Do not use ordinary plastic storage bags or formula bottle bags for storing expressed milk.

3. Use sealed and chilled milk within 24 hours if possible. Discard all milk that has been refrigerated more than 72 hours.

4. Freeze milk if you will not be using it within 24 hours. Frozen milk is good for at least 1 month (3 to 6 months if kept in a 0° freezer). Store it at the back of the freezer and never in the door section. Make sure to label the milk with the date it was frozen. Use the oldest milk first.

5. Freeze 2 to 4 ounces of milk per container (this is the average amount of a single feeding). You may also want to freeze some smaller amounts.

6. Do not add fresh milk to already frozen milk.

7. You can thaw the milk in the refrigerator, or you can thaw it more quickly by swirling the milk container in a bowl of warm water.

8. Do not use microwave ovens to heat bottles because they do not heat evenly. Uneven heating can easily scald the baby or damage the milk. Bottles can also explode if left in the microwave too long. Excess heat destroys important proteins and vitamins in the milk.

9.   Milk thawed in the refrigerator must be used within 24 hours.

10.   Do not refreeze your milk.

11.   Do not save milk from a used bottle for use at another feeding.

Weaning

There is no specific time to wean your baby. It depends entirely on the individual desires and needs of you and the baby. Either one of you can initiate the weaning process.

Some babies lose interest in breast-feeding between 9 and 12 months of age, or after they learn to drink from a cup. If you notice this starting to happen, do not try to force your baby to keep breast-feeding. Understand that this is not a rejection of you, but rather the first sign of your child's growing independence.

You may feel sad, guilty, lonely, or depressed about giving up the closeness and intimacy that comes from breast-feeding. These feelings are natural. Continue to cuddle and interact with your baby, and remember that weaning is a natural step in helping your child to grow up.

If you initiate weaning, you can wean your child first to a bottle and then to a cup, or directly to a cup. During weaning, you can express milk with which to feed your baby from the cup or bottle, or you can use infant formula. Formula does not provide all of the special nutrients and protective qualities that breast milk does, so it is generally best to breast-fed as long as possible.

If you choose to supplement breast-feeding with formula, you will still need to express milk in order to keep up your milk production and to keep your breasts from becoming engorged.

If you decide to use a bottle, introduce it gradually over several days. Start with one feeding per day. If the baby is extremely hungry when you first introduce the bottle, the baby may be more impatient. It may also help if another person introduces the bottle when you are not around. Many babies get upset if they are given a bottle when their mother is in the house; they may even refuse the bottle because they want to breast-feed instead. Do not force your baby to take a bottle. It may take time. Pressure to take a bottle may cause the baby to refuse the bottle completely.

After bottle-feedings have started, some babies may get frustrated when they breast-feed because the milk does not flow as fast from the breast as it does from a bottle.

The following suggestions may help:

❖ Select a bottle nipple with a slow flow.

❖ Pump for 1 to 2 minutes before you breast-feed.

❖ Massage the breast as you nurse to help the milk flow.

❖ Use relaxation techniques to enhance milk flow.

❖ Offer the breast before your baby gets overly hungry and becomes impatient.

Weaning to a cup has the following advantages over a bottle:

❖ It eliminates the step of weaning first to a bottle and then to a cup.

❖ Bottle-feeding for long periods of time or while sleeping can lead to tooth decay.

❖ Drinking from a bottle while lying flat can lead to middle ear infections.

❖ Prolonged bottle-feeding can lead to the bottle's becoming a security object, especially after the child is 1 year old.

Start with a trainer cup that has two handles and a snap-on lid with a spout, or use a small plastic glass. This will keep spills small while the baby is experimenting with holding the cup (and throwing it). Do not be surprised if the baby treats the cup as a plaything at first.

Offer breast milk in the cup, when available, starting once per day. It may be easiest to substitute a cup for breast-feeding at the midday feeding first, and the nighttime feeding last. Nighttime nursing is often a source of comfort and calming before going to sleep, and may be the hardest feeding to give up.

Be patient. Weaning is a gradual process, and it may take months before your baby is willing or able to take all liquids from a cup. Proceed gradually and let the baby's willingness and interest guide you. Once you have stopped breast-feeding entirely, your breasts will stop producing milk very quickly.

Until you and your baby develop a feeding routine, stay positive and try not to become discouraged. Remember, breast milk gives the baby more than just food. It also provides important antibodies to fight off infection, and it has medical and psychological benefits for both of you. Breast-feeding is the most natural gift that you can give your baby.

Appendix A:
Organizations to Contact
for Assistance

Antiepileptic Drug Pregnancy Registry
Massachusetts General Hospital
Harvard Medical School
Tel: 888-233-2334

Citizens United for Research in Epilepsy (CURE)
505 North Lake Shore Drive #4605
Chicago, IL 60611
CUREepi@aol.com
http://www.CUREepilepsy.org
Tel: 312-923-9117
Fax: 312-923-9118

Comprehensive Epilepsy Center
Boswell Building
300 Pasteur Drive
Stanford, CA
Tel: 650-725-6648

Epilepsy Foundation
4351 Garden City Drive, Suite 500
Landover, MD 20785-7223
http://www.epilepsyfoundation.org
Tel: 800-EFA-1000 (332-1000) or 301-459-3700
Fax: 301-577-2684

Chapters of the Epilepsy Foundation are located throughout the United
States. To find a chapter in your state, call the main Epilepsy Foundation
number and they will direct you to the chapter nearest to you.

Epilepsy Institute
257 Park Avenue South
New York, NY 10010
website@epilepsyinstitute.org
http://www.epilepsyinstitute.org
Tel: 212-677-8550
Fax: 212-677-5825

Family Caregiver Alliance
690 Market Street, Suite 600
San Francisco, CA 94104
info@caregiver.org
http://www.caregiver.org
Tel: 800-445-8106 or 415-434-3388
Fax: 415-434-3508

International Radiosurgery Support Association (IRSA)
P.O. Box 5186
Harrisburg, PA 17110
getinfo@irsa.org
http://www.irsa.org
Tel: 717-260-9808
Fax: 717-260-9809

National Association of Epilepsy Centers
5775 Wayzata Boulevard, Suite 200
Minneapolis, MN 55416
Tel: 888-525-6232 or 952-525-4526
http://www.naec-epilepsy.org

This site lists more than 60 specialized epilepsy centers across the United States and is an excellent source for finding a physician who specializes in treating epilepsy.

National Council on Patient Information and Education
4915 St. Elmo Avenue, Suite 505
Bethesda, MD 20814-6082
ncpie@ncpie.info
http://www.talkaboutrx.org
Tel: 301-656-8565
Fax: 301-656-4464

National Family Caregivers Association
10400 Connecticut Avenue, Suite 500
Kensington, MD 20895-3944
info@nfcacares.org
http://www.nfcacares.org
Tel: 800-896-3650 or 301-942-6430
Fax: 301-942-2302

National Institutes of Health (NIH) Neurological Institute
P.O. Box 5801
Bethesda, MD 20824
Tel: 800-352-9424 or 301-496-5751
http://www.ninds.nih.gov

National Organization for Rare Disorders (NORD)
P.O. Box 1968
55 Kenosia Avenue
Danbury, CT 06813-1968
orphan@rarediseases.org
http://www.rarediseases.org
Tel: 203-744-0100
Voice Mail: 800-999-NORD (999-6673)
Fax: 203-798-2291

Strong Epilepsy Center
601 Elmwood Ave, Box 673
Rochester, NY 14642
epilepsy@urmc.rochester.edu
Tel: 585-275-0698

Appendix B: The AED Pregnancy Registry

The Purpose of the Registry

Pregnant women generally avoid medications, but without antiepileptic drugs (AEDs), women with epilepsy are at risk of seizures. The AED Pregnancy Registry registers or enrolls women (over the telephone) who are pregnant and taking AEDs to participate in research. As more women register and report the outcomes of their pregnancies, researchers will be able to identify the safest AEDs to take during pregnancy and determine how safe each new AED is.

Who Should Participate

Any woman who is pregnant and taking AEDs can participate in the Pregnancy Registry. If you want to participate, call the registry early in your pregnancy (during the first trimester). You can still participate in the registry if you are already in your second or third trimester. The toll-free number for the registry is (888)233-2334. The registry coordinator will ask you questions such as your age, the date of your last menstrual period, and what AEDs and vitamins you are taking. By enrolling, you can give other women the best possible chance of a healthy pregnancy and a healthy baby. It will also help you with any future pregnancies you might have.

Enrolling in the registry takes very little time. Your initial phone call to the registry will take less than 10 minutes. At 7 months, there is another telephone interview that lasts approximately 5 minutes. There will be a brief 5-minute follow-up interview after your baby is born.

Confidentiality

The researchers at the registry understand that confidentiality is important. A coding system is used so that personal information, including your name and address, are not part of the registry database. No one who has participated in the registry will ever be identified.

Glossary

Abruptio placentae. A condition in which the placenta begins to detach itself from the wall of the uterus before the birth of the baby.

Absence seizure. A blank stare, beginning and ending abruptly; lasting only a few seconds; most common in children. You may also notice rapid blinking and some chewing movements of the mouth. The child or adult is unaware of what is going on during the seizure, but quickly returns to full awareness once it has stopped. It may result in learning difficulties.

Accidental hemorrhage. Vaginal bleeding usually indicates abruptio placentae; may be hidden for some time.

Alpha-fetoprotein. A protein produced by the fetus that is excreted into the amniotic fluid. Abnormal levels of alpha-fetoprotein may indicate brain or spinal cord defects, multiple fetuses, a miscalculated due date, or chromosomal disorders.

Amniocentesis. A common prenatal test in which a small sample of the amniotic fluid surrounding the fetus is removed and examined. It is often used during the second trimester of pregnancy (usually 15–18 weeks after a woman's last menstrual period) to rule out certain birth defects. Amniocentesis is the most common prenatal test used to diagnose chromosomal and genetic birth defects.

Amniotic sac. A thin-walled sac that surrounds the fetus during pregnancy.

Anemia. A condition that develops when blood is deficient in healthy red blood cells, the main transporter of oxygen to organs. If red blood cells are also deficient in hemoglobin, then the body is not getting enough iron. Symptoms of anemia, such as fatigue, occur because the organs are not getting enough oxygen. There are many types of anemia, all are very different in their causes and treatments. Iron-deficiency anemia, the most common type, is treatable with diet and iron supplements. Some forms of anemia, such as the anemia that develops during pregnancy, are even considered normal. Some types of anemia, however, may present lifelong health problems. Women in their childbearing years are particularly susceptible to iron-deficiency anemia because of the blood loss from menstruation and the increased blood supply demands during pregnancy. Certain forms of anemia are hereditary, and infants may be affected from the time of birth.

Antiepileptic drug (AED). A medication used to control epileptic seizures.

Astatic seizure. A seizure that causes sudden loss of muscle tension, in which the person falls down and is often injured.

Atonic seizure. A sudden loss of muscle tone that makes the person collapse and fall. In some people, all that happens is a sudden drop of the head. The person recovers and regains consciousness after a few seconds to a minute. Drop attacks can cause injuries because of the force of the fall.

Aura. Many people think an aura is a warning that a seizure may be imminent, but auras are actually the beginning of a seizure. Patients have described auras ranging from abnormal smells or tastes to a funny feeling in the stomach, and sounds, colors, or emotional rushes.

Automatism. Something a person does during a seizure in a state of diminished consciousness, such as pulling at clothing.

Birth defects. Malformations in the fetus. A birth defect may affect how the body looks, function, or both. It may be found before birth, at birth, or anytime after birth. Most defects are discovered within the first year of life. Some birth defects (cleft lip or clubfoot) are easy to see, but others (heart defects or hearing loss) are found using special tests (X-rays, CAT scans, echocardiography, or hearing tests). Birth defects can vary from mild to severe; some may cause the baby to die. Babies with birth defects may need surgery or other medical treatments, but with medical care they usually lead normal lives.

Blind trial. A drug trial in which neither subject nor doctor knows which treatment is being given, drug or placebo.

Braxton-Hicks contractions. Painless contractions during pregnancy that help the uterus to grow and the blood to circulate through the uterus.

Breech birth. An abnormal delivery presentation in which the baby's feet, knees, or buttocks come into the birth canal first, before the baby's head does.

Callosotomy. An operation for epilepsy that involves splitting the callosal body (split brain).

Carbamazepine (Tegretol). An excellent medication in its various forms that is mostly used for partial seizures. In general, it is very well tolerated and has some transient sedation effect, usually resolving in 3 days. Tegretol may cause myoclonic seizures and atypical absence seizures to worsen significantly. It may also cause a life-threatening blood count, liver dysfunction, and severe allergic rashes, including Steven Johnson's disease.

Cardiac defects. Atrial septal defect, tetralogy of Fallot, ventricular septal defect, coarctation of the aorta, patent ductus arteriosus, and pulmonary stenosis.

Cassette EEG (electroencephalography). A recording of long-term EEG by means of a tape recorder that can be hung on the belt.

Central nervous system (CNS). The brain and the spinal cord together form the central nervous system. The CNS is one division of the human nervous system.

Cervix. The lower part of the uterus that projects into the vagina; mostly fibrous tissue and muscle and circular in shape. During pregnancy, the cervix lengthens, serving as a barrier. When labor begins, the cervix begins to shorten, dilating to an opening of about 10 centimeters (4 inches) to allow the fetus to pass through. The cervix also thins and merges with the uterus (effacement) during the first stage of labor.

Cesarean section (C-section). The obstetric operation for delivering a baby through the abdominal wall. This is usually lower uterine segment cesarean section, or LSCS, carried out via a transverse cut in the lower part of the abdomen.

Chorionic villus. A test done during pregnancy to identify certain problems with the fetus. It is usually done when either of the parents has a family history of an inherited disease, or when the age of the mother (35 years old or older) increases her risk of having a baby with a chromosome defect. Chorionic villi are tiny finger-like projections found in the placenta. The genetic material in chorionic villus cells is identical to that in the fetal cells. During CVS, a sample of the chorionic villus cells is taken for biopsy. The general health of the fetus can be predicted by examining the chorionic villus cells for abnormalities. This procedure is usually done during the first 3 months of pregnancy, ideally between the eighth and twelfth weeks. CVS is not generally done after the twelfth week of pregnancy because increasing amounts of amniotic fluid make the procedure more difficult. Also, after 12 weeks it becomes more difficult to distinguish chorionic villus cells from the cells of the mother.

Chromosomes. The carriers of inherited predispositions; found in cell nuclei.

Cleft palate. A birth defect in which there is a split in the roof of the mouth.

Clonic seizures. A type of seizure that starts with a sudden cry, fall, and/or body stiffness followed by jerking movements as the muscles repeatedly tense and then relax. Skin may be bluish. Possible loss of bladder or bowel control as muscles relax. Usually lasts a minute or two, after which normal breathing returns. The person may be confused or tired afterwards, and fall into a deep sleep. Person may complain of sore muscles or bitten tongue upon awakening.

Clubfoot. A group of deformities of the ankles and feet or sometimes both. These defects are usually present at birth. The defect may be mild or severe, and may affect one or both of the ankles and/or feet. There are different forms of clubfoot. Some may include talipes equinovarus, when the foot is turned inward and downward; calcaneal valgus, when the foot is angled at the heel with the toes pointing upward and outward; metatarsus varus, when the front of the foot is turned inward. If not corrected, babies who are affected may develop an abnormal way of walking.

Colic. Strong abdominal pain, usually of fluctuating severity, with waves of pain seconds or a few minutes apart. Infantile colic is common among babies. It is caused by gas in the intestines, and is associated with feeding difficulties; colic is not dangerous.

Colostrum. Fluid in the breasts that nourishes the baby until breast milk becomes available. Colostrum contains fats, carbohydrates, white blood cells, protein, and antibodies.

Complex partial seizures. Complex and simple partial seizures are similar, but complex partial seizure is accompanied by impaired consciousness and recall. A person having a complex partial seizure will be unresponsive to questions or commands and will not be able to recall what happened during the seizure after it is over. Complex partial seizures used to be called temporal lobe or psychomotor seizures.

Cradle cap. A common condition in young babies in which crusty white or yellow scales form a "cap" on the scalp. Application of oil or a special shampoo usually helps to resolve this condition.

Diagnostic treatment. A trial treatment with antiepileptic medicine when it has not been possible to ascertain whether the person has epilepsy.

Down Syndrome. Named after John Langdon Down, the first physician to identify the syndrome, this is the most frequent genetic cause of mild to moderate mental retardation and associated medical problems; occurs in one out of 800 live births, in all races and economic groups. Down syndrome is a chromosomal disorder caused by an error in cell division that results in the presence of an additional third chromosome 21, or trisomy 21. To understand why Down syndrome occurs, the structure and function of the human chromosome must be understood. The human body is made up of cells that contain chromosomes, which are structures that transmit genetic information. Most cells of the human body contain 23 pairs of chromosomes, half of which are inherited from each parent. Only the human reproductive cells—the sperm cells in males and the ovum in females—have 23 individual chromosomes, not pairs. Scientists identify these chromosome pairs as the XX pair, present in females, and the XY pair, present in males, and number them 1 through 22.

Ectopic pregnancy. An abnormal pregnancy in which the fertilized egg implants outside of the uterus.

EDD.   Estimated due date.

EEG (electroencephalography).   A registration of the electrical activity of the brain using electrodes placed on the scalp.

Embryo.   The fetus is called an embryo during the first 8 weeks after conception.

Enzyme.   A substance that stimulates chemical processes.

Enzyme induction.   Stimulation of the liver's enzyme systems so that medicine and other substances are broken down faster than normally.

Epilepsy.   A group of disorders characterized by unprovoked, recurrent seizures—that is, sudden, transient disturbances of electrical activity in the brain—that disrupt normal neurologic functioning. Symptoms depend on the type of epilepsy and the location of the disturbance in the brain; epilepsy can include loss of consciousness, and motor, psychic, or sensory phenomena.

Epileptic focus.   An area in the brain that triggers epileptic activity.

Epileptic syndrome.   An age-linked type of epilepsy in which a group of different symptoms make up the picture.

Episiotomy.   An incision into the perineum (area of skin between the vagina and the anus) that is made during childbirth to enlarge the opening for delivery.

Ethosuxamide (Zarontin).   Medication that is good for absence seizures only; one of the safest anticonvulsants available. Hematological side effects and allergic reactions have been reported. Drowsiness, headaches, and abdominal pains may also occur.

Felbamate (Felbatol).   A very effective anticonvulsant, even for severe and resistant seizures such as Lenox-Gastaut syndrome, and generalized absence, myoclonic, and focal seizures. The use of felbamate is extremely limited, because of the severe and possibly fatal blood and liver damage associated with this medication.

Fetal alcohol syndrome. Birth defects caused by a mother's alcohol consumption during pregnancy. Children with the most severe effects have characteristic facial features (a small face, narrow eye openings, a short upturned nose, a flattened groove between the nose and the upper lip, and a thin upper lip), growth retardation, and mental and behavioral problems (central nervous system effects). They may also have birth defects that involve the eyes, ears, heart, urinary tract, and bones. Children with less severe effects may have one or a combination of these characteristics to a milder degree. Some experts use the term fetal alcohol spectrum disorder (FASD) to include all categories of alcohol effects on a fetus. When a pregnant woman drinks alcohol, the alcohol passes from her blood into the fetus. Large amounts of alcohol may damage fetal cells, especially those of the central nervous system. The exact way alcohol causes the damage is not known. From magnetic resonance imaging (MRI) and computed tomography (CT) scans of babies with FASD, it appears that alcohol may target specific areas of the developing brain.

Fetus. An unborn baby from the eighth week after conception until delivery.

Folate. Folate and folic acid are forms of a water-soluble B vitamin, occurring naturally in food. Folic acid is the synthetic form of this vitamin that is found in supplements and fortified foods. A key observation of researcher Lucy Wills nearly 70 years ago led to the identification of folate as the nutrient needed to prevent the anemia of pregnancy. Dr. Wills demonstrated that anemia could be corrected by a yeast extract. Folate was identified as the corrective substance in yeast extract in the late 1930s, and was first extracted from spinach leaves in 1941. Folate is necessary for the production and maintenance of new cells. This is especially important during periods of rapid cell division and growth such as infancy and pregnancy. Folate is needed to make DNA and RNA, the building blocks of cells. It also helps make normal red blood cells and prevents anemia; prevents birth defects.

GABA (Gamma-amino butyric acid). An inhibitory neurotransmitter.

Gabapentin (Neurontin). An anticonvulsant medication design to mimic the GABA molecule. GABA is an inhibitory neurotransmitter; theoretically, increasing GABA concentration decreases brain excitation and stops seizures. Taking GABA alone (available in health food stores) is useless, because GABA does not cross the blood-brain barrier; Neurontin was designed to have a GABA structure, yet be able to penetrate into the brain. It is a very safe anticonvulsant, but its efficacy is questionable. High doses are needed to achieve good seizure control. Side effects include dizziness and drowsiness. Other uses have been found for Neurontin, including the treatment of migraines (as a preventative agent), neuropathies, and trigeminal neuralgia. The actual mechanism of action of this medication is unknown, but it clearly is not what it was originally designed to be.

Gastric tone.   Determines the sensitivity of the stomach to distention.

Generalized seizure.   A seizure in which the abnormal electrical activity involves the whole brain.

Generalized tonic-clonic seizure (grand mal seizures).   During this type of seizure, the person falls to the ground, the entire body stiffens, and the person's muscles begin to jerk or spasm (convulse).

Gestational diabetes.   A type of diabetes that begins during pregnancy in which the body is not able to use the sugar (glucose) in the blood as well as it should, resulting in a high level of sugar in the blood. Gestational diabetes affects about 4% of all pregnant women. It usually begins in the fifth or sixth month of pregnancy (between 24 and 28 weeks). Gestational diabetes usually goes away after the baby is born.

Half-life.   The time it takes for the concentration of a drug to fall to half of its peak concentration; important in finding out how many doses should be taken in a day.

Hemoglobin.   The substance in red blood cells that carries oxygen.

Human chorionic gonadotropin.   A hormone produced by the placenta about 10 days after fertilization.

Hyperventilation.   Rapid breathing; used as a method of provocation during EEG. Particularly suited to provoke absences.

Hypsarrhythmia.   Special changes in EEG in infantile spasms.

Ictal. That which happens during a seizure.

Idiopathic epilepsy. Epilepsy with no known cause; hereditary factors combined with biochemical changes in the brain may be involved.

Informed consent. A person's agreement to participate in a scientific investigation after being told the relevant facts and risks involved.

Intensive monitoring. Registration by cassette or video EEG.

Interictal. That which happens between seizures.

Jaundice. A condition in which the skin and whites of the eyes are yellowish in color.

Kegel exercises. Strengthen the pelvic-floor muscles; done regularly during pregnancy and after childbirth; can help prevent leakage of urine, as well as increase sexual responsiveness.

Klonopin (clonazepam). A benzodiazepine that is similar to Valium; may be helpful for myoclonic, generalized, and partial seizures. It may also be helpful for infantile spasms or Lenox-Gastaut syndrome. Side effects are mostly related to sedation, drooling, cognitive impairment, and hyperactivity.

Lamotrigine (Lamictal). An effective, well-tolerated medication good for generalized and partial seizures that may also be effective for absence seizures, atomic seizures, and Lenox-Gastaut syndrome. It may be associated with the development of a severe rash, especially if combined with valproic acid. Studies indicate that the rash does not occur frequently if the dose is gradually titrated upwards. Other side effects are mild, and consist mostly of dizziness, drowsiness, or headaches.

Levetiracetam (Keppra). An effective adjunct medication for partial seizure control; no serious side effects have been reported. It has been used in practice since 2000; in June 2005 it was approved for use in children 4 years of age and older. For resistant partial seizures, however, this medication should be attempted before resorting to invasive managements.

Lobes. The brain can be divided down the middle lengthwise into two halves called the cerebral hemispheres. Each hemisphere of the cerebral cortex is divided into four lobes by various sulci and gyri. The sulci (or fissures) are the grooves, and the gyri are the bumps that can be seen on the surface of the brain. The folding of the cerebral cortex produced by these bumps and grooves increases the amount of cerebral cortex that can fit in the skull. Although most people have the same patterns of gyri and sulci on the cerebral cortex, no two brains are exactly alike.

Lumbar puncture. Puncture of the lumbar spine with a thin needle.

Mastitis. Inflammation of the breast, usually caused by bacterial infection via damaged nipples.

Myoclonic jerk. A sudden jerk of the arm or leg that can occur as a particular seizure type in epilepsy. Many people experience something similar when falling asleep, but it is not epilepsy.

Myoclonic seizures. Sudden brief, massive muscle jerks that may involve the whole body or parts of the body. May cause the person to spill what they were holding or fall off a chair.

Neuron. A nerve cell.

Neurotransmitter. A chemical substance that allows the passing of neural impulses from cell to cell.

Oxcarbazepine. The generic name for the antiepileptic drug Trileptal, an excellent, safe anticonvulsant. It is very similar to carbamazepine (Tegretol) in structure, but designed to have the epoxide moiety. The epoxide is the part of carbamazepine responsible for drowsiness, severe allergic reactions, and liver damage and blood dyscrasia that may cause fatal side effects. The seizure control obtained with Trileptal is as good and in some situations better than with Tegretol. Side effects are minor, and may cause some temporary drowsiness, mild allergic reaction, and decreased sodium level in the elderly. In short, Trileptal is an improved Tegretol, more effective and better tolerated; it has never been the cause of any fatal side effects.

Partial seizure. A seizure that occurs only in a specific part of brain. Partial seizures often start with an aura; usually arising in the frontal or temporal lobe. The symptoms of a partial seizure depend on area of the brain involved in the seizure.

Pharmacokinetics. The study of the time course of drug and metabolite levels in different fluids, tissues, and excreta of the body, and of the mathematical relationships required to develop models to interpret such data.

Phenobarbital. A drug for generalized and partial seizures that may be used for febrile seizures; more frequently used during the neonatal period, but rarely used after 5 years of age because of its potential to cause learning difficulties. Side effects include hyperactivity and other behavioral difficult-ies in about half of the children treated (aged 2 to 10). Drowsiness and rashes may also occur. Rare impairments of liver functions and blood counts have been reported. Phenobarbital is best tolerated in children less than 1 year old.

Phenytoin (Dilantin, Phenytek). Medication most effective in partial sei-zures, but also good for generalized seizures and status epilepticus. It is also helpful for the control of seizures that occur on an intermittent basis. Phenytoin causes many side effects, including hypertrophy (swelling) of the gums, coarsening of facial features, facial hair growth, and brain atrophy over extended use. It may also cause the usual side effects, including allergic reaction, and blood count and liver enzyme dysfunction. The allergic reaction may be severe (Steven Johnson's disease) and life-threatening.

Photosensitive epilepsy. A form of epilepsy in which seizures can be caused by blinking light.

Placebo. Tablets (often called chalk tablets or sugar pills) that have no medicinal content and therefore no physiologic effect (often used in blind studies.)

Plasma volume. The volume of plasma in the blood. Plasma, the noncellu-lar portion of blood, consists of water, inorganic salts (such as sodium, potassium, and calcium), and organic molecules (such as sugars and pro-teins). Normal plasma volume in an average adult is usually 3 liters, while total blood volume is about 5 liters.

Placenta.   An organ shaped similar to a flat cake that grows in the uterus during pregnancy; provides for metabolic interchange between the fetus and mother.

Polycystic ovary syndrome (PCOS).   A hormonal imbalance condition in which normal, regular ovulation does not occur. This hormonal imbalance also affects other body systems, such as metabolism and the cardiovascular system. The cause of PCOS is not fully known; occurs in 5% to 10% of women ages 20 to 40.

Polytherapy.   A treatment involving more than one medication.

Premature.   Born before full term, or 37 weeks, of gestation.

Preterm labor.   A typical full-term pregnancy lasts 37 to 42 weeks, calculated from the first day of the last menstrual period to childbirth. Preterm labor, or premature labor, is the early onset of uterine contractions before 37 weeks, but after 20 weeks of pregnancy.

Primidone (Mysoline).   Mysoline is the same as phenobarbital; metabolizes to phenobarbital plus PEMA. It causes more sedation than phenobarbital, and may be helpful in some seizures that are poorly controlled with phenobarbital.

Prodromes.   Longer prewarning of a seizure, often lasting several days; most commonly depression.

Prognosis.   The expected future course of an illness.

Pseudo seizure.   A seizure that is caused by psychic factors (not epilepsy).

Psychogenic seizure.   Unplike epileptic seizures, psychogenic seizures are not the result of an abnormal electrical discharge from the brain, but rather a physical manifestation of a psychological disturbance. They are a type of conversion disorder that is usually involuntary.

Secondary generalization.   A partial seizure that develops into a generalized seizure.

Simple partial seizures.   A seizure during which the person is alert and able to respond to questions or commands. People who have had a simple partial seizure can remember what occurred during the seizure.

Slow-release formula. A special form of medicine that can be taken fewer times a day with the same effect.

SPECT (single photon emission computerized tomography) scanning. An investigation of the blood flow in the brain.

Spike. A particular wave pattern in EEG that is typical of epilepsy.

Spina bifida. Malformation of the spinal cord and spine.

Spinal cord. An enlarged collection of nerve fibers and nerve cell bodies that exits the skull and travels through the vertebrae of the spine.

Spinal fluid. Fluid that surrounds the brain and the spinal cord.

Status epilepticus. A seizure that lasts longer than 30 minutes, or a series of seizures with no recovery of consciousness or behavioral functions between attacks. Partial seizures can progress to status epilepticus.

Steady state. The situation arising when the blood concentration remains the same from day to day.

Stereotypy. Meaningless repeated movements typical during complex partial seizures.

Stillbirth. Delivery of a dead baby after the 20th week of pregnancy and birth; loss of a fetus before the 20th week of pregnancy is considered a miscarriage.

Stress convulsions. Generalized seizures triggered by stress.

Symptom. A sign of illness.

Symptomatic epilepsy. Epilepsy in which the cause is known.

Synapse. A space in the brain where two nerve cells interact.

Syndrome. A collection of symptoms that together make up an illness.

Teratogenic drug. A drug that can cause birth defects if given to a pregnant woman or if she gets pregnant while she is taking it.

Therapeutic range.   The concentration of medication in the blood that is the most effective with the fewest side effects.

Tiagabine (Gabitril).   A medication that blocks the reuptake of GABA in the synaptic area to be metabolized, therefore increasing GABA concentration and reducing brain excitation. Used primarily as an adjunct for partial seizures, but may be effective in other seizure types as well. Generally well tolerated; has never been reported to cause serious side effects. Unfortunately, it has a poor effect on infantile spasm treatment and cannot be a substitute to Sabril as originally hoped.

Todd's paralysis.   Brief or transient focal weakness after a seizure.

Tolerance development.   The reduced effect of medicine over time.

Tonic convulsions.   Convulsions with muscular rigidity.

Tonic seizure.   A seizure in which the muscles suddenly contract and stiffen, often causing the person to fall down (another form of "drop attack").

Tonus.   Muscular tension.

Topiramate (Topamax).   Another excellent AED with multiple mechanisms of action. Good for focal and generalized seizures; found helpful with Lenox-Gastaut syndrome, infantile spasm, and other seizure types. Generally very well tolerated; may cause a decrease in the appetite and psychosis. At times, it may also be associated with a temporary sedative effect. For some children it may be the only medication that can completely control frequent intractable seizures.

Trimester.   One of three phases of pregnancy, each lasting 3 months.

Ultrasound.   A method of imaging the fetus and the female pelvic organs using high-frequency sound waves, which bounce off body structures.

Umbilical cord.   A cord that connects the fetus to the placenta; contains two arteries and a vein, which carry oxygen and nutrients to the fetus and waste products away from the fetus.

Uterine wall.   The wall of the uterus.

Uterus. Also called the womb, the uterus is a hollow, pear-shaped organ located in a woman's lower abdomen between the bladder and the rectum; the fertilized egg becomes implanted in the wall of the uterus.

Valproic acid (Depakene). An excellent anticonvulsant for generalized and focal seizures. Recently it has started to be used for nonconvulsive disorders, including migraine prevention and as a mood stabilizer for bipolar disorders. Valproic acid comes in Depakene and Depakote forms. Seizures controlled with this medication include myoclonic seizures, absence seizures, and mixed-type seizures. Side effects include initial transient sedation and abdominal pain (better tolerated with the Depakote form). It may also increase the appetite (causing weight gain), cause some transient hair loss (which improves with zinc supplementation), or cause liver and blood count abnormalities, although this is rare. Hyperammonemia and pancreatic dysfunction have also been reported. In children younger than 3, and especially younger than 2, valproic acid may cause a severe fatal liver disease in a frequency as high as 1 in 300. Many patients taking valproic acid may have an associated carnitine deficiency. Carnitine can be supplemented with Carnitor syrup or tablets.

Varicose veins. Twisted, enlarged veins near the surface of the skin; can occur anywhere there is increased pressure in a vein close to the skin, but most commonly in the legs and ankles. Varicose veins do not usually cause any symptoms. When there are symptoms, they are often worse after prolonged sitting or standing, or late in the day.

Video EEG. A long-term EEG in which a video recording of a person is combined with an EEG recording. The video EEG monitoring test is a more specialized form of an EEG test in which the patient is constantly monitored over a video screen. This allows doctors to observe brain-wave activity during the time a seizure or spell is occurring in order to determine the most effective way to treat the condition. The test requires admission to the hospital for 3 to 5 days.

Vigabatrin (Sabril). An AED that is unavailable in the United States because it can cause irreversible changes in visual fields. It is still a very important medication because of its beneficial effect in infantile spasms. It has been shown to stop severe seizures in three out of four children who have tuberous sclerosis and infantile spasms. It is associated with a much less adverse reaction compared to ACTH (the standard treatment for infantile spasms). Sabril is one of the GABA designer medications, and the only one that effectively does what it was designed to do. Sabril blocks the degradation of GABA by blocking the effect of the enzyme GABA transaminase, thus increasing GABA concentration in the presynaptic area. Other side effects of Sabril include psychosis (rare), and some mild fatigue or gastrointestinal upset, which are related.

Wada test.   An investigation to find out in which half of the brain the speech center is located. The Wada test consists of behavioral testing after the injection of an anesthetic (such as sodium amobarbital or sodium methohexital) into the right or left internal carotid artery. The activities of one of the cerebral hemispheres are temporarily suspended, so the abilities subserved by the other hemisphere can be tested in isolation. Typical uses of the test include the lateralization of language abilities and a determination that the person will not be amnesic after surgery. Epilepsy surgery is usually performed for non-life-threatening conditions, making this an important consideration.

Water breaking.   The rupture of the amniotic sac; usually occurs at the onset of labor.

Wharton's jelly.   Accumulations of jelly sometimes seen on the umbilical cord, which are of no consequence.

Yeast infection (Candida albicans).   A common vaginal infection, especially during pregnancy; characterized by itching, redness, and a white discharge.

Zarontin.   See ethosuximide

Zonisamide (Zonegran).   Zonegran is effective for the treatment of both partial and generalized seizures. It is very effective in absence seizure control, and may be substituted for Depakote in some of the absence seizures resistant to Zarontin, or in those who have both absence and generalized convulsive seizures. Generally well tolerated, but may cause extreme drowsiness in some people. Zonegran may cause some rare but serious hematological side effects.

Bibliography

Abbasi F, Krumholz A, Kittner SJ, et al. Effects of menopause on seizures in women with epilepsy. *Epilepsia.* 1999;40:205–210.

ACOG educational bulletin. Seizure disorders in pregnancy. No. 231, December 1996. Committee on Educational Bulletins of the American College of Obstetricians and Gynecologists. *Int J Gynecol Obstet.* 1997;56:279–286.

Adab N, Jacoby A, Smith D, et al. Additional educational needs in children born to mothers with epilepsy. *J Neurol Neurosurg Psych.* 2001;70:15–21.

American Academy of Neurology. Quality Standards Subcommittee. Practice parameter: management issues for women with epilepsy (summary statement). *Neurology.* 1998;51:944–948.

American Academy of Pediatrics. The transfer of medications and other chemicals into human milk. *Pediatrics.* 1994;93:137–150.

Annegers JF, Hauser WA, Elveback LR, et al. Congenital malformations and seizure disorders in the offspring of parents with epilepsy. *Int J Epidemiol.* 1978;7:241–247.

Ardinger HH, Atkin JF, Blackston RD, et al. Verification of the fetal valproate syndrome phenotype. *Am J Med Genet.* 1988;29:171–185.

Beastall GH, Cowan RA, Gray JMB, et al. Hormone binding globulins and anticonvulsant therapy. *Scott Med J.* 1985;30:101–105.

Beaussart-Deaye J, Bastin N, Demarcq C. *Epilepsies and Reproduction.* Vol. 2. Grine Lille, France: Nord Epilepsy Research and Information Group; 1986:72.

Beck-Managetta G, et al. Malformations and minor anomalies in children of epileptic mothers: Preliminary results of the prospective Helsinki study. In: Janz D, Dam M, Richens A, eds. *Epilepsy, Pregnancy, and the Child.* New York, NY: Raven; 1982:317–323.

Ben-Shlomo I, Franks S, Adashi EY. The polycystic ovary syndrome: nature or nurture? *Fertil Steril.* 1995;63:953–954.

Bilo L, Meo R, Valentino R, et al. Abnormal pattern of luteinizing hormone pulsatility in women with epilepsy. *Fertil Steril.* 1991;55:705–711.

Biton V, Mirza W, Montouris G, et al. Weight change associated with valproate and lamotrigine monotherapy in patients with epilepsy. *Neurology.* 2001;56:172–177.

Bogliun G, Beghi E, Crespi V, et al. Anticonvulsant medications and bone metabolism. *Acta Neurol Scand.* 1986;74:284–288.

Brann DW, Hendry LB, Mahesh VB. Emerging diversities in the mechanism of action of steroid hormones. *J Steroid Biochem Mol Biol.* 1995;52:113–133.

Buehler BA, Delimont D, Van Waes M, et al. Prenatal prediction of risk of the fetal hydantoin syndrome. *N Engl J Med.* 1990;322:1567–1572.

Centers for Disease Control and Prevention. Recommendations for the use of folic acid to reduce the number of cases of spina bifida and other neural tube defects. *MMWR.* 1992;41(RR-14):1–7.

Chang S, Ahn C. Effects of antiepileptic drug therapy on bone mineral density in ambulatory epileptic children. *Brain Dev.* 1994;16:382–385.

Clayton RN, Ogden V, Hodgkinson J, et al. How common are polycystic ovaries in normal women and what is their significance for the fertility of the population? *Clin Endocrinol.* (Oxf) 1992;37:127–134.

Commission on Genetics, Pregnancy, and the Child, International League Against Epilepsy. Guidelines for the care of women of childbearing age with epilepsy. *Epilepsia.* 1993;34:588–589.

Coulam CB, Annegers JF. Do oral anticonvulsants reduce the efficacy of oral contraceptives? *Epilepsia.* 1979;20:519–526.

Craig J, Morrison P, Morrow J, et al. Failure of periconceptional folic acid to prevent a neural tube defect in the offspring of a mother taking sodium valproate. *Seizure.* 1999;8:253–254.

Cummings SR, Nevitt MC, Browner WS, et al. Risk factors for hip fracture in white women. Study of Osteoporotic Fractures Research Group. *N Engl J Med.* 1995; 332:767–773.

Daly LE, Kirke PN, Molloy A, et al. Folate levels and neural tube defects: implications for treatment. *JAMA.* 1995;274:1698–1702.

Dana-Haeri J, Oxley J. Reduction of free testosterone by antiepileptic medications. *Br Med J.* 1982;284:85–86.

Dana-Haeri J, Trimble MR, Oxley J. Prolactin and gonadotrophin changes following generalized and partial seizures. *J Neurol Neurosurg Psychiatry.* 1983;46:331–335.

Dansky L, Andermann E, Roseblatt D, et al. Anticonvulsants, folate levels and pregnancy outcome. *Ann Neurol.* 1987;21:176–182.

Dansky LV, Andermann E, Andermann F. Marriage and fertility in epileptic patients. *Epilepsia.* 1980;21:261–271.

Delgado-Escueta AV, Janz D. Consensus guidelines: preconception counseling, management, and care of the pregnant women with epilepsy. *Neurology.* 1992;42(4 suppl 5):149–160.

DiLiberti JH, Farndon PA, Dennis NR, et al. The fetal valproate syndrome. *Am J Med Genet.* 1984;19:473–481.

Dravet C, Julian C, Legras C, et al. Epilepsy, antiepileptic medications, and malformations in children of women with epilepsy: a French prospective cohort study. *Neurology.* 1992;42(4 suppl 5):75–82.

Drislane FW, Coleman AE, Schomer DL, et al. Altered pulsatile secretion of luteinizing hormone in women with epilepsy. *Neurology.* 1994;44:306–310.

Fenwick PBC, Mercer C, Grant R, et al. Nocturnal penile tumescence and serum testosterone levels. *Arch Sex Behav.* 1986;15:13–21.

Finn DA, Gee KW. The estrous cycle, sensitivity to convulsants and the anticonvulsant effect of a neuroactive steroid. *J Pharmacol Exp Ther.* 1994;271:164–170.

Finn DA, Roberts AJ, Crabbe JC. Neuroactive steroid sensitivity in withdrawal seizure-prone and resistant mice. *Alcoholism Clin Exp Res.* 1995;19:410–415.

Finnell RH, Buehler BA, Kerr BM, et al. Clinical and experimental studies linking oxidative metabolism to phenytoin-induced teratogenesis. *Neurology.* 1992;42:25–31.

Finnell RH. Genetic differences in susceptibility to anticonvulsant drug induced developmental defects. *Pharmacol Toxicol.* 1991;69:223–227.

Fisher RS, Vickrey BG, Gibson P, et al. The impact of epilepsy from the patient's perspective I. Descriptions and subjective perceptions. *Epilepsy Res.* 2000;41:39–51.

Friis ML. Facial clefts and congenital heart defects in children of parents with epilepsy: genetic and environmental etiologic factors. *Acta Neurol Scand.* 1989;79:433–459.

Gaily E, Granstrom ML. Minor anomalies in children of mothers with epilepsy. *Neurology.* 1992;42(suppl 5):128–131.

Gaily E, Granstrom ML, Hiilesmaa V, et al. Minor anomalies in offspring of epileptic mothers. *J Pediatr.* 1988;112:520–529.

Gaily EK, Granstrom ML, Hiilesmaa VK, et al. Head circumference in children of epileptic mothers: contributions of drug exposure and genetic background. *Epilepsy Res.* 1990;5:217–222.

Gaily E, Kantola-Sorsa E, Granstrom ML. Intelligence of children of epileptic mothers. *J Pediatr.* 1988;113:677–684.

Gaily E, Kantola-Sorsa E, Granstrom ML. Specific cognitive dysfunction in children with epileptic mothers. *Dev Med Child Neurol.* 1990;32:403–414.

Gordon N. Folate metabolism and neural tube defects. *Brain Dev.* 1995;17:307–311.

Gough H, Goggin T, Bissessar A, et al. A comparative study of the relative influence of different anticonvulsant medications, UV exposure and diet on vitamin D and calcium metabolism in outpatients with epilepsy. *Q J Med.* 1986;59:569–577.

Gustavson EE, Chen H. Goldenhar syndrome, anterior encephalocele, and aquaductal stenosis following fetal primidone exposure. *Teratology.* 1985;32:13–17.

Hanson JW, Smith DW. The fetal hydantoin syndrome. *J Pediatr.* 1975;87:285–290.

Harden CL, Pulver MC, Ravdin L, et al. The effect of menopause and perimenopause on the course of epilepsy. *Epilepsia.* 1999;40:1402–1407.

Haukkamaa M. Contraception by Norplant subdermal capsules is not reliable in epileptic patients on anticonvulsant treatment. *Contraception.* 1986;33:559–565.

Hauser WA, Annegers JF, Kurland LT. Incidence of epilepsy and unprovoked seizures in Rochester, Minnesota: 1935–1984. *Epilepsia.* 1993;34:453–468.

Hauser WA, Hesdorffer DC. Risk factors. In: Hauser WA, Hesdorffer DC, eds. *Epilepsy: Frequency, Causes and Consequences.* New York, NY: Demos Medical Publishing; 1990:53–100.

Herzog AG. Reproductive endocrine considerations and hormonal therapy for women with epilepsy. *Epilepsia.* 1991;32(suppl 6):527–533.

Herzog AG. Progesterone therapy in women with complex partial and secondary generalized seizures. *Neurology.* 1995;45:1660–1662.

Herzog AG. Progesterone therapy in women with epilepsy: a 3-year follow-up. *Neurology.* 1999;52:1917–1918.

Herzog AG, Klein P, Ransil BJ. Three patterns of catamenial epilepsy. *Epilepsia.* 1997;38:1082–1088.

Herzog AG, Seibel MM, Schomer DL, et al. Reproductive endocrine disorders in women with partial seizures of temporal lobe origin. *Arch Neurol.* 1986;43:341–346.

Hernandez-Diaz S, Werler MM, Walker AM, et al. Folic acid antagonists during pregnancy and the risk of birth defects. *N Engl J Med.* 2000;343:1608–1614.

Hill RM, Vernaiud WM, Retting GM, et al. Relationship of antiepileptic drug exposure of the infant and developmental potential. In: Janz D, Dam M, Richens A, eds. *Epilepsy, Pregnancy, and the Child.* New York, NY: Raven; 1982.

Holmes GL, Kloczko N, Weber DA, et al. Anticonvulsant effect of hormones on seizures in animals. In: Porter RJ, Mattson RH, Ward AM Jr, Dam M, eds. *Advances in Epileptology: XVth Epilepsy International Symposium.* New York, NY: Raven Press; 1984:265–268.

Holmes LB, Harvey EA, Coull BA, et al. The teratogenicity of anticonvulsant medications. *N Engl J Med.* 2001;344:1132–1138.

Hom AC, Buterbaugh GG. Estrogen alters the acquisition of seizures kindled by repeated amygdala stimulation or pentylenetetrazol administration in ovariectomized female rats. *Epilepsia.* 1986;27:103–108.

Isojarvi JIT, Laatikainen TJ, Pakarinen AJ, et al. Polycystic ovaries and hyperandrogenism in women taking valproate for epilepsy. *N Engl J Med.* 1993;329:1383–1388.

Isojarvi JIT, Rattya J, Myllyla VV, et al. Valproate, lamotrigine, and insulin-mediated risks in women with epilepsy. *Ann Neurol.* 1998;43:446–451.

Jager-Roman E, Deichl A, Jakob S, et al. Fetal growth, major malformations, and minor anomalies in infants born to women receiving valproic acid. *J Pediatr.* 1986; 108:997–1004.

Jones KL, Lacro RV, Johnson KA, et al. Pattern of malformations in the children of women treated with carbamazepine during pregnancy. *N Engl J Med.* 1989; 320:1661–1666.

Knochenhauer ES, Key TJ, Kahsar-Miller M, et al. Prevalence of the polycystic syndrome in unselected black and white women of the southeastern United States: a prospective study. *J Clin Endocrinol Metab.* 1998;83:3078–3082.

Koch HV, Kraft D, von Herrath D. Influence of diphenylhydantoin and Phenobarbital on intestinal calcium transport in the rat. *Epilepsia.* 1972;13:829–834.

Koch S, Loesche G, Jager-Roman E, et al. Major birth malformations and antiepileptic medications. *Neurology.* 1992;42(suppl 5):83–88.

Koch S, Titze K, Zimmerman RB, et al. Long-term neuropsychological consequences of maternal epilepsy and anticonvulsant treatment during pregnancy for school-age children and adolescents. *Epilepsia.* 1999;40:1237–1243.

Krauss GL, Brandt J, Campbell M, et al. Antiepileptic medication and oral contraceptive interactions: a national survey of neurologists and obstetricians. *Neurology.* 1996;46:1534–1539.

Kruse K, Suss A, Busse M, et al. Monomeric serum calcitonin and bone turnover during anticonvulsant treatment and in congenital hypothyroidism. *J Pediatr.* 1987; 111:57–63.

Landgren S, Backstrom T, Kalistratov G. The effect of progesterone on the spontaneous interictal spike evoked by the application of penicillin to the cat's cerebral cortex. *J Neurol Sci.* 1976;36:119–133.

Laurence KM, James N, Miller MH, et al. Double-blind, randomized controlled trial of folate treatment before conception to prevent the recurrence of neural tube defects. *Br Med J.* 1981;282:1509–1511.

Lindhout D, Omtzigt JC, Cornel MC. Spectrum of neural-tube defects in 34 infants prenatally exposed to antiepileptic medications. *Neurology.* 1992;42(4 suppl 5): 111–118.

Lindhout D, Omtzigt JG. Teratogenic effects of antiepileptic medications: implications for the management of epilepsy in women of childbearing age. *Epilepsia.* 1994; 35(suppl 4):S19–28.

Lindhout D, Schmidt D. In-utero exposure to valproate and neural tube defects. *Lancet.* 1986;1:1392–1393.

Lobo RA. A disorder without identity: "HCA," "PCO," "PCOD," "PCOS," "SLS." What are we to call it?! *Fertil Steril.* 1995;63:158–160.

Loughnan PM, Gold H, Vance JC. Phenytoin teratogenicity in man. *Lancet.* 1973;1(794):70–72.

Luhdorf K. Endocrine function and antiepileptic treatment. *Acta Neurol Scand.* 1983;67(suppl 94):15–19.

Marcus EM, Watson CW, Goldman PL. Effects of steroids on cerebral electrical activity: epileptogenic effects of conjugated estrogens and related compounds in the cat and rabbit. *Arch Neurol.* 1966;15:521–532.

Martin PJ, Millac PA. Pregnancy, epilepsy, management and outcome: a 10-year perspective. *Seizure.* 1993;2:277–280.

Mattson RH, Cramer JA, Caldwell BV, et al. Treatment of seizures with medroxyprogesterone acetate: preliminary report. *Neurology.* 1984;34:1255–1258.

Mattson RH, Cramer JA, Collins JF, et al. Comparison of carbamazepine, Phenobarbital, phenytoin, and primidone in partial and secondarily generalized tonic-clonic seizures. *N Engl J Med.* 1985;313:145–151.

Mattson RH, Cramer JA, Darney PD, et al. Use of oral contraceptives by women with epilepsy. *JAMA.* 1986;256:238–240.

McAuley JW, Anderson GD. Treatment of epilepsy in women of reproductive age: pharmacokinetic considerations. *Clin Pharmacokinet.* 2002;41:559–579.

McEwen BS. Multiple ovarian hormone effects on brain structure and function. *J Gend Specif Med.* 1998;1:33–41.

Meo R, Bilo L, Nappi C, et al. Derangement of the hypothalamic GnRH pulse generator in women with epilepsy. *Seizure.* 1993;2:241–252.

Milunsky A, Jick H, Jick SS, et al. Multivitamin/folic acid supplementation in early pregnancy reduces the prevalence of neural tube defects. *JAMA.* 1988;262:2847–2852.

Miranda AF, Wiley MJ, Wells PG. Evidence for embryonic peroxidase-catalyzed bioactivation and glutathione-dependent cytoprotection in phenytoin teratogenicity: modulation by eicosatetraynoic acid and buthione sulfoximine in murine embryo culture. *Toxicol Appl Pharmacol.* 1994;124:230–241.

Morrell MJ, Flynn KL, Seale CG, et al. Reproductive dysfunction in women with epilepsy: antiepileptic drug effects on sex-steroid hormones. *CNS Spectrums.* 2001; 6:771–786.

Morrell MJ, Guidice L, Flynn KL, et al. Predictors of ovulatory failure in women with epilepsy. *Ann Neurol.* 2002;52:704–711.

Morrell MJ, Guldner GT. Self-reported sexual function and sexual arousability in women with epilepsy. *Epilepsia.* 1996;37:1204–1210.

Morrell MJ, Sarto GE, Osborne Shafer P, et al. Health issues for women with epilepsy: a descriptive survey to assess knowledge and awareness among healthcare providers. *J Women's Health Gend Based Med.* 2000;9:959–965.

Morrell MJ, Sperling MR, Stecker M, et al. Sexual dysfunction in partial epilepsy: a deficit in physiologic sexual arousal. *Neurology.* 1994;44:243–247.

Morrell MJ. Effects of epilepsy on women's reproductive health. *Epilepsia.* 1998;39(suppl 8):S32–37.

Morrell MJ. Sexuality in epilepsy. In: Engel J, Pedley TA, eds. *Epilepsy: A Comprehensive Textbook.* New York, NY: Lippincott-Raven; 1997:2021–2026.

Mulinare J, Corder JF, Erickson JD, et al. Periconceptional use of multivitamins and the occurrence of neural tube defects. *JAMA.* 1988;260:3141–3145.

Murialdo G, Galimberti CA, Gianelli MV, et al. Effects of valproate, phenobarbital, and carbamazepine on sex steroid setup in women with epilepsy. *Clin Neuropharmacol.* 1998;21:52–58.

Murialdo G, Galimberti CA, Magri F, et al. Menstrual cycle and ovary alterations in women with epilepsy on antiepileptic therapy. *J Endocrinol Invest.* 1997;20:519–526.

Nau H, Tzimas G, Mondry M, et al. Antiepileptic medications alter endogenous retinoid concentration: a possible mechanism of teratogenesis of anticonvulsant therapy. *Life Sci.* 1995;57:53–60.

Odlind V, Olsson SE. Enhanced metabolism of levonorgestrel during phenytoin treatment in a woman with Norplant implants. *Contraception.* 1986;33:257–261.

Ogawa Y, Kaneko S, Otani K, et al. Serum folic acid levels in epileptic mothers and their relationship to congenital malformations. *Epilepsy Res.* 1991;8:75–78.

Oguni M, Dansky L, Andermann E, et al. Improved pregnancy outcome in epileptic women in the last decade: relationship to maternal anticonvulsant therapy. *Brain Dev.* 1992;14:371–380.

Omtzigt JGC, Los FJ, Grobee DE, et al. The risk of spina bifida aperta after first-trimester exposure to valproate in a prenatal cohort. *Neurology.* 1992;42(suppl 5):119–125.

Pearlman MD, Tintinalli JE, Lorenz RP. Blunt trauma during pregnancy. *N Eng J Med.* 1990;323:1609–1613.

Perrucca E. Clinical implications of hepatic microsomal enzyme induction by antiepileptic medications. *Pharmacol Ther.* 1987;33:139–144.

Pfaff DW, McEwen BS. Actions of estrogens and progestins on nerve cells. *Science.* 1983;219:808–814.

Practice parameter: management issues for women with epilepsy (summary statement). Report of the Quality Standards Subcommittee of the American Academy of Neurology. *Neurology.* 1998;51:944–948.

Recommendations for the use of folic acid to reduce the number of cases of spina bifida and other neural tube defects. *MMWR Recomm Rep.* 1992;41:1–7.

Reinisch JM, Sanders SA, Mortensen EL, et al. In utero exposure to phenobarbital and intelligence deficits in adult men. *JAMA.* 1995;274:1518–1525.

Robert E, Guibaud P. Maternal valproic acid and congenital neural tube defects [Letter]. *Lancet.* 1982;2:937.

Rosa FW. Spina bifida in infants of women treated with carbamazepine during pregnancy. *N Engl J Med.* 1991;324:674–677.

Rudd NL, Freedom RM. A possible primidone embryopathy. *J Pediatr.* 1979;94:835–837.

Samuels P. Neurologic disorders. In: Gabbe SG, Niebyl JR, Simpson JL, Annas GJ, eds. *Obstetrics: Normal and Problem Pregnancies.* 3rd ed. New York, NY: Churchill-Livingstone; 1996:1135–1154.

Sato Y, Kondo I, Ishida S, et al. Decreased bone mass and increased bone turnover with valproate therapy in adults with epilepsy. *Neurology.* 2001;57:445–449.

Schmidt D, Beck-Mannagetta G, Janz D, et al. The effect of pregnancy on the course of epilepsy: a prospective study. In: Janz D, Dam M, Richens A., eds. *Epilepsy, Pregnancy and the Child.* New York, NY: Raven Press; 1982;39–49.

Schupf N, Ottman R. Likelihood of pregnancy in individuals with idiopathic/cryptogenic epilepsy: social and biologic influence. *Epilepsia.* 1994;35:750–756.

Schupf N, Ottman R. Reproduction among individuals with idiopathic/cryptogenic epilepsy: risk factors for reduced fertility in marriage. *Epilepsia.* 1996;37:833–840.

Schupf N, Ottman R. Reproduction among individuals with idiopathic/cryptogenic epilepsy: risk factors for spontaneous abortion. *Epilepsia.* 1997;38:824–829.

Seip M. Growth retardation, dysmorphic facies and minor malformations following massive exposure to phenobarbitone in utero. *Acta Paediatr Scand.* 1976;65:617–621.

Sheth R, Wesolowski C, Jacob J, et al. Effect of carbamazepine and valproate on bone mineral density. *J Pediatr.* 1996;127:256–262.

Shuster EA. Epilepsy in women. *Mayo Clin Proc.* 1996;71:991–999.

Sperling MR, Pritchard PB, Engel J, et al. Prolactin in partial epilepsy: an indicator of limbic seizures. *Ann Neurol.* 1986;20:716–722.

Spiegel E, Wycis H. Anticonvulsant effects of steroids. *J Lab Clin Med.* 1945;30:947–953.

Steegers-Theunissen RPM, Renier WO, Borm GF, et al. Factors influencing the risk of abnormal pregnancy outcome in epileptic women: a multicentre prospective study. *Epilepsy Res.* 1994;18:261–269.

Stitt SL, Kinnard WJ. The effect of certain progestins and estrogens on the threshold of electrically induced seizure patterns. *Neurology.* 1968;18:213–216.

Strickler SM, Dansky LV, Miller MA, et al. Genetic predisposition to phenytoin-induced birth defects. *Lancet.* 1985;2:746–749.

Takeshita N, Seino Y, Ishida H, et al. Increased circulating levels of gamma-carboxyglutamic acid-containing protein and decreased bone mass in children on anticonvulsant therapy. *Calcif Tissue Int.* 1989;44:80–85.

Tauboll E, Lindstrom S. The effect of progesterone and its metabolite 5-alpha-pregnan-3-alpha-ol-20-one on focal epileptic seizures in the cat's visual cortex in vivo. *Epilepsy Res.* 1993;14:17–30.

Teramo K, Hiilesmaa V, Brady A, et al. Fetal heart rate during a maternal grand mal epileptic seizure. *J Perinatal Med.* 1979;7:3–6.

Thomas J, McLean JH. Castration alters susceptibility of male rats to specific seizures. *Physiol Behav.* 1991;49:1177–1179.

Thorp JA, Gaston L, Caspers DR, et al. Current concepts and controversies in the use of vitamin K. *Medications.* 1995;49:376–387.

Tomson T, Lindbom U, Sundqvist A, et al. Red cell folate levels in pregnant epileptic women. *Eur J Clin Pharmacol.* 1995;48:305–308.

Valimaki M, Tiihonen M, Laitinen K, et al. Bone mineral density measured by dual-energy x-ray absorptiometry and novel markers of bone formation and resorption in patients on antiepileptic medications. *J Bone Miner Res.* 1994;9:631–637.

Van Allen M, Fraser FC, Dallaire L, et al. Recommendations on the use of folic acid supplementation to prevent the recurrence of neural tube defects. *Can Med Assoc J.* 1993;149:1239–1243.

Vernillo AT, Rifkin BR, Hauschka PV. Phenytoin affects osteoblastic secretion from osteoblastic rat osteosarcoma 17/2.8 cells in culture. *Bone.* 1990;11:309–312.

Verrotti A, Greco R, Morgese G, et al. Increased bone turnover in epileptic patients treated with carbamazepine. *Ann Neurol.* 2000;47:385–388.

Wallace H, Shorvon S, Tallis R. Age-specific incidence and prevalence rates of treated epilepsy in an unselected population of 2,052,922 and age-specific fertility rates of women with epilepsy. *Lancet.* 1998;352:1970–1973.

Webber MP, Hauser WA, Ottman R, et al. Fertility in persons with epilepsy:1935–1974. *Epilepsia.* 1986;27:746–752.

Weinstein RS, Bryce GF, Sappington LJ, et al. Decreased serum ionized calcium and normal vitamin D metabolite levels with anticonvulsant drug treatment. *J Clin Endocrinol Metab.* 1984;58:1003–1009.

Werler MM, Shapiro S, Mitchell AA. Periconceptional folic acid exposure and risk of occurrent neural tube defects. *JAMA.* 1993;269:1257–1261.

Wooley DE, Timiras PS. Estrous and circadian periodicity and electroshock convulsions in rats. *Am J Physiol.* 1962;202:379–382.

Wooley DE, Timiras PS. The gonad-brain relationship: effects of female sex hormones and electroshock convulsions in the rat. *Endocrinology.* 1962;70:196–209.

Woolley CS, Schwartzkroin PA. Hormonal effects on the brain. *Epilepsia.* 1998; 39(suppl 8):S2–S8.

Woolley CS, Weiland NG, McEwen BS, et al. Estradiol increases the sensitivity of hippocampal CA1 pyramidal cells to NMDA receptor-mediated synaptic input: correlation with dendritic spine density. *J Neurosci.* 1997;17:1848–1859.

Yates JRW, Ferguson-Smith MA, Shenkin A, et al. Is disordered folate metabolism the basis for the genetic predisposition to neural tube defects? *Clin Genet.* 1987; 31:279–287.

Yerby M. Treatment of epilepsy during pregnancy. In: Wyllie E, ed. *The Treatment of Epilepsy*, 2nd ed. Baltimore, Md: Williams & Wilkins; 1996:785–798.

Yerby M, Koepsell T, Daling J. Pregnancy complications and outcomes in a cohort of women with epilepsy. *Epilepsia.* 1985;26:631–635.

Yerby M, Morrell MJ. Efficacy, safety and tolerability of zonisamide in women. Sexual dysfunction and hormonal abnormalities in women with epilepsy. *Epilepsia.* 2000; 41(suppl 7):199.

Yerby MS. Epilepsy and pregnancy: new issues for an old disorder. *Neurol Clin.* 1993;11:777–786.

Yerby MS, Friel PN, McCormick K, et al. Pharmacokinetics of anticonvulsants in pregnancy: alterations in plasma protein binding. *Epilepsy Res.* 1990;5:223–228.

Yerby MS, Friel PN, McCormick K. Antiepileptic drug disposition during pregnancy. *Neurology.* 1992;42(4 suppl 5):12–6.

Zahn CA, Morrell MJ, Collins SD, et al. Management issues for women with epilepsy: a review of the literature. American Academy of Neurology Practice Guidelines. *Neurology.* 1998;51.

Index